OXFORD MEDICAL PUBLICATIONS

Stroke Care

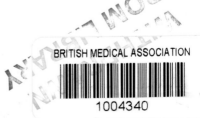

Published and forthcoming Oxford Care Manuals

Cardiovascular Disease in the Elderly: A Practical Manual
Rosaire Gray and Louise Pack

Dementia Care: A Practical Manual
Jonathan Waite, Rowan H Harwood, Ian R Morton, and David J Connelly

Diabetes Care: A Practical Manual
Rowan Hillson

Headache: A Practical Manual
David Kernick and Peter J Goadsby (eds)

Motor Neuron Disease: A Practical Manual
Kevin Talbot, Martin R Turner, Rachael Marsden, and Rachel Botell

Multiple Sclerosis Care: A Practical Manual
John Zajicek, Jennifer Freeman, and Bernadette Porter (eds)

Neuromuscular Disorders in the Adult: A Practical Manual
David Hilton-Jones, Jane Freebody, and Jane Stein

Preventive Cardiology: A Practical Manual
Catriona Jennings, Alison Mead, Jennifer Jones, Annie Holden, Susan Connolly, Kornelia Kotseva, and David Wood

Stroke Care: A Practical Manual (2nd Edition)
Rowan H. Harwood, Farhad Huwez, and Dawn Good

Stroke Care: A practical manual

SECOND EDITION

Rowan H. Harwood

Consultant Physician
Nottingham University Hospitals
Nottingham, UK

Farhad Huwez

Consultant Physician
Lead Stroke Services
Basildon and Thurrock University Hospital
Basildon, UK

Dawn Good

Clinical Stroke Service Specialist
Nottingham University Hospitals
Nottingham, UK

OXFORD
UNIVERSITY PRESS

OXFORD
UNIVERSITY PRESS

Great Clarendon Street, Oxford OX2 6DP

Oxford University Press is a department of the University of Oxford.
It furthers the University's objective of excellence in research, scholarship,
and education by publishing worldwide in

Oxford New York

Auckland Cape Town Dar es Salaam Hong Kong Karachi
Kuala Lumpur Madrid Melbourne Mexico City Nairobi
New Delhi Shanghai Taipei Toronto

With offices in

Argentina Austria Brazil Chile Czech Republic France Greece
Guatemala Hungary Italy Japan Poland Portugal Singapore
South Korea Switzerland Thailand Turkey Ukraine Vietnam

Oxford is a registered trade mark of Oxford University Press
in the UK and in certain other countries

Published in the United States
by Oxford University Press Inc., New York

British Library Cataloguing in Publication Data
Data available

Library of Congress Cataloging-in-Publication-Data
Data available

Typeset by Glyph International, Bangalore, India
Printed in Great Britain
on acid-free paper by
Ashford Colour Press Ltd., Gosport, Hampshire

ISBN 978–0–19–955831–5

10 9 8 7 6 5 4 3 2 1

Foreword

Recent years have seen several books about stroke, but *Stroke care: A practical manual* remains an important guide to the practical day to day management of stroke patients. The success of the book is reflected in this second edition, which retains the simple, informative, and user friendly style of the previous edition but has been updated to include new information, guidelines, and practices. It is an excellent 'what to', 'how to', and 'when to' guide that appeals to a multidisciplinary audience and is relevant to all practitioners involved in stroke care.

The management of stroke patients and its prevention have come a long way in the last two decades following revolutionary changes in imaging of the brain and blood vessels, the introduction of thrombolysis, and new strategies in rehabilitation. Stroke has been prioritized in many countries, leading to restructuring of stroke services and a plethora of guidelines often varying in recommendations. There also remain several unknowns in stroke care, especially as earlier management and more comprehensive imaging or investigations throw up new challenges and many therapeutic strategies remain to be backed up by robust clinical evidence. This book is aimed at guiding clinicians through many of the commonly encountered situations in stroke, interpreting available evidence and guidelines in the context of day to day patient care. Each chapter deals sympathetically with important aspects of care in the different phases of patients' journey through their pathway of care, starting at the hyperacute end and covering long-term and palliative care.

The simple and engaging style of the book and the wealth of practical information will give pleasure to the readers and help them to deliver better quality of care to stroke patients.

Lalit Kalra, PhD, FRCP
Professor of Stroke Medicine
Clinical Neurosciences Division
King's College London
London, UK

Preface

Stroke medicine is maturing as a discipline, and evidence, policy, and practice are ever changing. A book of practical advice needs constant reconsideration, updating, and revision. We have been much encouraged by the reception of the first edition of this book, and we welcome the chance to offer a second edition.

The book is written for people who look after stroke patients, in particular, doctors, nurses, and therapists working in stroke units. A new staff member may find it useful to read through the book, but mainly it is a book to refer back to.

Our main text is direct and directive (you might say dogmatic). If you are faced with a clinical problem, you need to know what do, not about the uncertainties of academic debate. We are well aware of the need to justify bold assertions with high-quality evidence, but the quality of evidence we have available is variable. Statements that lack the backing of a randomized controlled trial are both uncertain, and vulnerable to change.

However, the randomized trial is not the only type of evidence. We try to capture some of the accumulated wisdom about how to do things that resides in an experienced and functioning team. Much of our advice is based on experience, or what we have been taught, illuminated by hard evidence where it is available, or where sensible extrapolations can be made from what is known. You might want to follow-up the evidence for what we suggest, but that is not our main purpose. We present key pieces of evidence in a fairly raw form in boxes scattered throughout the text. We confine references to these boxes. We doubt that any more would be used much, and we are not trying to compete with more encyclopaedic reference texts or electronic searching.

We follow a time-based sequence of chapters, which follows the journey of a stroke patient from diagnosis to outcome. We take a very broad view of what stroke care requires. We are writing from the perspective of general internal and geriatric medicine rather than as specialist neurologists. We struggle most when working at the limits of our knowledge and experience. In this book we push at the boundaries of the subject. For example, the quality of clinical decision making is very topical, has made an appearance in postgraduate examinations, and we spend large amounts of clinical time working on difficult decisions. Therefore, we include a chapter on it. Many stroke patients die, so we include a chapter on terminal care. We are unaware of any other written guidelines on how to discharge a patient. Advice on managing undiagnosed coma, pain, or disturbed behaviour is not specific to stroke, but are all issues which frequently arise in our own stroke practices.

There is some repetition. Some issues arise early and persist (such as positioning, venous thrombosis prophylaxis, and continence). The distinction between acute and rehabilitation care is blurred. Secondary prevention starts early rather than at the end of the process as our chapter order suggests. Hopefully each section is fairly self-contained, but we cross reference where possible.

This is a book of guidelines. Guidelines are intended to give help and advice, but are not a substitute for proper professional assessment and opinion. Evidence changes with time, interpretation of evidence may vary with circumstances and from individual to individual, and different places have quite justifiably different ways of doing things. We have checked drug doses, but correct prescription remains the responsibility of the prescriber, who may need to take account of local policies or guidelines. Similarly, on legal and ethical issues, we write from the perspective of the law and current practice in England and Wales, but hope that the general principles will be of interest and use elsewhere.

Since the first edition our colleague and friend Peter Berman has died. He was a wise, knowledgeable, and perceptive pragmatist, who read the entire text of the first edition and made many helpful suggestions. He also did much to advance stroke medicine in the UK. In writing the first edition we also took advice from a number of others, whose contribution we continue to acknowledge: Vincent Crosby, Leela Duari, John Gladman, Tony Goddard, Miles Humberstone, Tim Jaspan, Roger Knaggs, Charlotte Morton, Jan Riley, Nina Squires, Udayaraj UmaSankar, and Mark Willmot. Adrian Blundell, Amlyn Evans, Kay Gaynor, Clare Gordon, Naseer Haboubi, Suzanne Hawkins, Becca O'Brien, Julie Phillips, Kate Radford, and Jane Terry have helped us with the second edition. Dr Sami Khan, consultant neuroradiologist, Basildon Hospital, contributed some of the magnetic resonance images. We are very grateful to them all. Mistakes are our own.

We must also thank our patients and their families, who inspire us to pursue stroke medicine as a 'defined speciality', requiring organized care by a team that has interest and expertise. We would like to dedicate this book to them, and to the memory of Peter Berman.

Contents

Detailed contents

Symbols and abbreviations

📖	cross reference
🖰	website
ACE	angiotensin-converting enzyme
ACEI	angiotensin-converting enzyme inhibitor
ADL	activities of daily living
AF	atrial fibrillation
AFO	ankle–foot orthosis
AIM	activate–initiate–monitor
AMT	Abbreviated Mental Test
APTT	activated partial thromboplastin time
ARB	angiotensin receptor blocker
ASPECTS	Alberta stroke program early CT score
AVM	arteriovenous malformation
AVPU	Alert, rousable to Voice, rousable to Pain, Unconscious
bd	twice a day
CADASIL	cerebral autosomal dominant arteriopathy with subcortical infarcts and leukoencephalopathy
CCB	calcium channel blocker
CHD	coronary heart disease
CI	confidence interval
CIMT	constraint-induced movement therapy
CNS	central nervous system
CPR	cardiopulmonary resuscitation
CPSP	central poststroke pain
CSF	cerebrospinal fluid
CT	computed tomography
CTA	computed tomography angiography/angiogram
DIC	disseminated intravascular coagulation
DNAR	do not attempt resuscitation
DSM-IV	Diagnostic and Statistical Manual of the American Psychiatric Association, fourth revision
DVT	deep vein thrombosis
DWI	diffusion-weighted imaging
ECG	electrocardiogram
ECST	European Carotid Surgery Trial
ESR	erythrocyte sedimentation rate

FAST	Face Arm and Speech Test
FBC	full blood count
FDP	fibrin degradation product
FES	functional electrical stimulation
FMD	fibromuscular dysplasia
GCS	Glasgow Coma Scale
GI	gastrointestinal
GKI	glucose–potassium–insulin
GP	general practitioner
Hb	haemoglobin
HMGCoA	hydroxymethylglutaryl-coenzyme A
HRT	hormone replacement therapy
ICH	intracerebral haemorrhage
IM	intramuscular
INR	international normalized ratio
IQR	interquartile range
IST	International Stroke Trial
ITT	intention to treat
IV	intravenous
LACI	lacunar infarct
LDL-C	low-density lipoprotein-cholesterol
LMN	lower motor neuron
LMWH	low-molecular-weight heparin
MAL	Motor Activity Log
MCA	middle cerebral artery
MELAS	mitochondrial encephalomyopathy with lactic acidosis and stroke-like episodes
MMSE	Mini-Mental State Examination
MR	modified release
MRA	magnetic resonance angiogram/angiography
MRI	magnetic resonance image/imaging
mRS	modified Rankin Scale
MRSA	methicillin-resistant *Staphylococcus aureus*
NICE	National Institute of Health and Clinical Excellence
NIH	National Institutes of Health
NINDS	National Institute of Neurological Disorders and Stroke
NNT	number needed to treat
O_2	oxygen
OCSP	Oxfordshire Community Stroke Project
OR	odds ratio
OT	occupational therapist

PACI	partial anterior circulation infarct
PCA	posterior cerebral artery
PCC	prothrombin complex concentrate
PEG	percutaneous endoscopic gastrostomy
PFO	patent foramen ovale
PIN	personal identification number
PO	by mouth
POCI	posterior circulation infarct
PR	via the rectum
qds	four times a day
RCT	randomized controlled trial
RIG	radiologically-guided gastrostomy
RR	relative risk
SAH	subarachnoid haemorrhage
SaO_2	arterial haemoglobin oxygen saturation
SC	subcutaneous
SIADH	syndrome of inappropriate secretion of antidiuretic hormone
SLE	systemic lupus erythematosus
SLT	speech and language therapy
SNRI	serotonin and norepinephrine reuptake inhibitor
SSRI	selective serotonin reuptake inhibitor
SSS	Scandinavian Stroke Score
TACI	total anterior circulation infarct
tds	three times a day
TENS	transcutaneous electrical nerve stimulation
TIA	transient ischaemic attack
tPA	tissue plasminogen activator
UK	United Kingdom
UMN	upper motor neuron
WFNS	World Federation of Neurological Surgeons
WHO	World Health Organization

Chapter 1

Is it a stroke?

Presentation of stroke

A diagnosis is an explanation, in biological terms, of a problem that a patient presents. An accurate diagnosis allows you to:
- Initiate specific treatments (and avoid worthless ones).
- Give an explanation of what is going on to the patient and others.
- Indicate chances of recovery and recurrence.

Stroke is a syndrome—a collection of symptoms and signs—which are usually obvious. The established WHO definition is:

> *a rapidly developing episode of focal or global neurological dysfunction, lasting longer than 24 hours or leading to death, and of presumed vascular origin.*

This definition has limitations:
- Some patients who appear to have had a stroke, have something other than cerebral infarction or haemorrhage (sometimes called 'stroke mimics').
- Neurological deficit progresses to some extent over the first 24h in about 25% of cases, and deterioration within the first week is common.
- It tells us nothing about the underlying pathology. More precise characterization of the type of stroke gives us clues about treatment options, prognosis, and risk of recurrence.
- If thrombolysis is being considered for acute stroke, 'time is brain'. Treatment must be delivered without delay, and no later than within 4.5h of symptom onset. Work-up must therefore begin without waiting to see if the deficit will resolve spontaneously—although in the face of rapidly resolving symptoms, administering potentially dangerous treatment would be unwise.
- Some non-specific presentations (immobility, falls, confusion, or incontinence) may be due to vascular brain disease, amongst other things.
- Comorbid conditions (especially in elderly people) can make diagnosis difficult.
- A number of cerebrovascular conditions fall outside the definition, including vascular dementia, silent infarction on brain imaging, and transient ischaemic attack (TIA).
- Subarachnoid haemorrhage fits the clinical definition for a stroke, but behaves and is managed as a separate entity.

An alternative definition of stroke is:

> *focal brain injury caused by sudden interruption of blood flow.*

Whilst accurate, this definition relies on the results of imaging, and includes some patients with transient symptoms. For practical clinical purposes it offers no great advantage.

What else might it be?

Transient ischaemic attack

(See also 📖 Neurovascular or TIA clinics, p.274.)

A TIA is an acute, focal, loss of cerebral function, or transient monocular blindness (amaurosis fugax), of presumed vascular origin, but the symptoms last <24h.

- Initially it is indistinguishable from a stroke.
- Most TIAs last less than an hour. It is difficult to define a lower limit to duration. Some descriptions say 'seconds', and 5% last less than a minute in published series, but it is difficult to imagine nerve cell failure due to ischaemia and recovery in much less than a minute. There may be problems with patients' recall of the passage of time when anxious.
- Amaurosis fugax is a rapidly progressive loss of vision, or partial loss of vision, in one eye (often, but not exclusively, 'like a curtain coming down'), coming on over a few seconds to a minute. After a variable time, usually seconds to a few minutes, it resolves with gradual recovery of vision over the whole visual field.
- Hemiplegic migraine is excluded.
- The main difficulty is making an accurate diagnosis based only on the history, and the absence of examination or investigation findings that suggest another diagnosis. Considerable uncertainty may remain.
- The importance of TIA and minor stroke lies in their propensity to recur: 10% in a week, 20% in a month. A third of these recurrences are persisting, disabling, or fatal strokes. Patients with TIA and minor stroke should be offered thorough and rapid investigation, and appropriate secondary prevention.
- Risk factors, and prognosis for stroke recurrence and ischaemic heart disease, are identical for TIA and minor stroke, regardless of symptom duration. However, higher and lower risk situations can be defined for individuals according to what symptoms, risk factors, and investigation findings they have (e.g. see 📖 Box 10.22, p.276 and 📖 Recurrence, p.286).
- About a quarter of patients with clinical TIA have an appropriate infarct on computed tomography (CT) brain imaging, half on diffusion-weighted magnetic resonance imaging (MRI) (including most of those in whom symptoms last over an hour). However, imaging evidence of infarction does not change management.
- Transient dizziness, confusion, vertigo, double vision, syncope, and drop attacks should not be diagnosed as TIA in the absence of other neurological findings.

Other differential diagnoses

- From the perspective of hospital admissions, about 25% of patients referred with possible stroke have something else.
- Some uncertainty is inevitable, but experienced doctors are better at diagnosing (and ruling out) stroke than less experienced ones.
- Mimics are most likely to be referred as possible stroke where there is cognitive impairment, loss of consciousness or seizure at onset, an inexact time of onset, an absence of focal neurological signs or symptoms, or an inability to classify the stroke to a typical location (e.g. using the Oxfordshire Community Stroke Project (OCSP) classification).

- Important differential diagnoses are shown in Table 1.1. Others that may arise include Bell's palsy, psychiatric illnesses, multiple sclerosis, metabolic disturbances, intoxication, transient global amnesia, dementia, and Parkinson's disease.
- Ask a neurologist's opinion if you are struggling to explain the clinical features, or are considering some of the more difficult or rare diagnoses.

Table 1.1 Conditions that can cause stroke-syndrome ('stroke-mimics')

Diagnosis	Key features
Old stroke, with increased weakness during intercurrent illness	Old neurological signs are often worse during intercurrent illnesses, especially infections, or appear to be so. Excluding a recurrent stroke is difficult, but rapid return to previous level of function is usual with appropriate treatment. Diffusion-weighted MRI is the best way to make a definite diagnosis of new stroke
Fits, with Todd's paresis	Commonest cause for misdiagnosis of recurrent stroke. Clinical diagnosis, usually requiring an eyewitness. Consider ictal features (loss of consciousness, convulsions, tongue biting, incontinence) and postictal features (headache, sleepiness, confusion). Diffusion-weighted MRI is the best way to make a definite diagnosis of new stroke
Cerebral tumours, primary or secondary	CT scan diagnosis. There may be features of raised intracranial pressure (headache, vomiting, drowsiness, papilloedema). Onset is slower than stroke. A stepwise progression over days or weeks is associated with space-occupying lesions, but only 1 in 6 patients with a progressive course has a tumour. Onset may be sudden if there is bleeding into a tumour
Hypoglycaemia	Almost always drug-induced, severe, hypoglycaemia. Usually rapidly reversible, but hemiplegia can persist ≥24h
Subdural haematoma	CT scan diagnosis. If significant, will cause drowsiness. Sometimes headache, confusion, hemiplegia or aphasia. Features may fluctuate
Cerebral abscess	CT scan diagnosis. Usually due to spread from sinuses or ear. Onset is subacute, but not always with prodromal infective symptoms. Headache usual. Later drowsiness, vomiting, delirium, and bradycardia. Aphasia, visual field defects, and facial weakness more common than hemiplegia. Avoid lumbar puncture. Needs surgical drainage. 25% mortality, even if optimally treated
Encephalitis	May sometimes be confused with stroke. 15% have focal signs. Usually mild preceding febrile illness, headache and drowsiness. Sometimes fits, confusion and gradual-onset coma. Ophthalmoplegia, nystagmus, other cranial nerve, cerebellar, and sensory signs possible. Neck may not be stiff. CT scan may be normal. CSF usually abnormal

Table 1.1 (Contd.)

Diagnosis	Key features
Cerebral vasculitis	Difficult to diagnose. Primary or secondary (to temporal arteritis, amphetamines, cocaine, SLE, infection, etc.). Can result in infarct or bleed. Headache prominent, focal neurological deficits include cranial nerve palsies or delirium. ESR can be raised, but this and other systemic markers will typically be normal in a primary CNS vasculitis. MRI and CSF abnormal. Check autoantibodies. May need angiography or temporal artery/brain/meningeal biopsy. Treat underlying cause and/or high-dose steroids
Venous thrombosis	Difficult to diagnose. Most have headache, half have raised intracranial pressure (nausea, papilloedema), some have focal neurological signs (hemiparesis or paraplegia) or fits. May be secondary to thrombophilia, trauma, infection, or postpartum. CSF is often abnormal (raised pressure, high protein, few red and white cells). CT may show hyperdensity of cortical veins or sinuses, filling defects with contrast (empty delta sign), infarction, disproportionate swelling, and haemorrhage. MR or CT venography is usually diagnostic
Conversion disorder	Lack of cranial nerve findings, neurological findings in a nonvascular distribution, inconsistent examination

Features prompting caution include:
- Headache (25% of patients with infarcts have a headache, usually mild).
- Pyrexia.
- Malaise or prodromal illness.
- Gradual progression over days.
- Features of raised intracranial pressure (headache, worst at night, on waking, and on coughing; drowsiness; vomiting; hypertension with bradycardia; papilloedema).
- Young age, or absence of vascular risk factors.
- Unobtainable or uncertain history.

Some transient neurological conditions can mimic TIA. These include:
- ***Migraine with aura*** The aura, usually a visual disturbance starting in one homonymous hemifield, develops over 5–30min, and lasts <1h. Visual phenomena include lights, halos, ziz-zag lines, scotomata or hemianopias, which can expand across the entire vision. Paraesthesia, limb heaviness, or hemiparesis develop in up to 40%, with or after visual symptoms, but rarely in isolation. They spread progressively across body parts (hand to arm to face) over several minutes, slower than TIA or sensory seizures. Aphasia can occur. Headache, usually unilateral and throbbing, typically starts as the aura is resolving, lasts 4–72h, with nausea, photo- and phonophobia, and worse with movement. Side may vary with attacks. Aura may occur without headache

(in 3–5% of migraineurs, increasing with age), during or after the headache, and may last >24h. Basilar territory symptoms are possible (vertigo, ataxia, dysarthria). Retinal migraine comprises recurrent attacks of monocular visual loss in younger adults, without headache, starting as enlarging scotomata, lasting minutes to an hour.

- *Fits* Generalized seizures imply loss of consciousness. The patient is rigid and may become blue during the attack. May be followed by uni-lateral weakness (Todd's paresis, lasting a few hours to a day). Partial seizures start in clear consciousness, but may be secondarily general-ized. They may be motor or sensory, with jerking or tingling that builds up and spreads. Complex partial seizures comprise a disturbance of content of consciousness, with sensory hallucinations (smell or taste, remembered scenes or déjà vu, distorted perceptions of the world), and motor features such as chewing or organized motor activity like undressing. Aphasia may occur. 2% of patients with stroke have a seizure at onset, half generalized and half partial.

- *Syncope* presents with loss of consciousness and postural tone due to a sudden fall in cerebral blood flow. The patient is pale, sweaty, clammy and floppy. Light-headedness may occur before syncope with dimming or loss of vision. A third have amnesia for the event.

- *Transient global amnesia* Middle aged or elderly people. Sudden onset. Loss of memory for new information (anterograde amnesia), may also be retrograde amnesia (past events). No loss of personal identity (patients know who they are), problem solving, language, or visuospatial orientation. Look healthy and repetitively ask the same questions. May have headache. Good recovery, recurrence is rare.

Differential diagnosis of coma

- Stroke will sometimes result in sustained unconsciousness (especially when due to bleeding, very large infarcts, or some basilar artery terri-tory strokes). Exclude other causes of coma (metabolic, infective), as some are treatable (Table 1.2).
- Impaired consciousness results from:
  - Bilateral cerebral cortical disease (hypoxic, metabolic, toxic, infec-tive, epileptic).
  - Impairment of brainstem reticular activating system (lesions of mibrain to midpons, or compression from transtentorial herniation due to supra- or infratentorial pressure).
- Large cerebral infarcts with oedema increase intracranial pressure enough to impair cortical function bilaterally, or cause tentorial hernia-tion (e.g. see 🕮 Fig. 2.1, p.45).
- Evaluation and treatment must be rapid, and must proceed together.
- Look for asymmetry—in tone, movement, and reflexes, and test braistem function (pupillary light reflex, doll-eye manoeuvre, corneal and gag reflexes).
- If the pupils are symmetrically reactive, and there are no focal neuro-logical signs, the coma is probably toxic or metabolic in origin.

- Coma developing over seconds to minutes suggests a cardiovascular, cerebrovascular, or epileptic cause. If there was recent trauma, consider extradural or subdural haematoma.
- Drug abuse is a cause of otherwise unexplained coma.
- Neurological clues help localization (Table 1.3). But remember that anticholinergic drugs and anoxia can produce large pupils, while opiates and some metabolic disorders give small pupils (usually reactive).
- Anyone in coma needs an immediate CT head scan—unless you are sure of the diagnosis, or that the patient would not have wanted intervention.

Table 1.2 Differential diagnosis of coma

Cause	Clues
Metabolic	
Hypoglycaemia	Glucometer
Diabetic ketoacidosis or hyperosmolar coma	Glucometer, acidosis, ± ketonuria
Hyper- or hyponatraemia	Serum sodium
Hypo- or hyperthermia	Temperature
Hepatic, uraemic coma	Stigmata, flap, history, blood tests
Septic encephalopathy	Fever, white count, inflammatory markers, focal signs or tests
Myxoedema coma /thyroid storm	History, clinical state, thyroid function tests
Hypoxia/hypercapnoea	History, pulse oximetry, arterial blood gases
Toxic	
Opiate poisoning	History, constricted pupils, response to naloxone
Benzodiazepines	History, response to flumazenil
Other drug poisoning (alcohol, tricyclics, phenothiazines)	Smell, tachycardia, agitation, hyper-reflexia, dilated pupils, blood alcohol.
Drugs of abuse	History, blood or urine toxicology
Carbon monoxide poisoning	Carboxy-haemoglobin (usually >40% to produce coma)
Trauma	
Head injury	History, external signs, CT scan
Shock	
Cardiogenic, pulmonary embolus, hypovolaemic, septic, anaphylactic, drug-induced, addisonian, neurogenic	Pulse, BP, peripheral perfusion, urine output

Table 1.2 *(Contd.)*

Cause	Clues
Tropical infections	
Malaria, typhoid, rabies, trypanosomiasis	Recent travel, temperature, blood tests
Neurological	
Fits, status epilepticus, post-convulsive	History, convulsions, EEG
Cerebral infarction/primary intracerebral haemorrhage/ sub-arachnoid haemorrhage	History, signs, CT scan
Subdural or extradural haematoma	History of trauma. CT scan. Lucid interval after injury
Meningitis, encephalitis	Fever, malaise, headache, neck and skin signs, CT, lumbar puncture
Hypertensive encephalopathy	BP, fundi, headache, confusion, urinalysis, renal function
Brain tumour, abscess	CT scan

Table 1.3 Localizing the cause of coma

Level	Features
Infra-tentorial	Brainstem causes usually have the most obvious signs and are easiest to diagnose.
	Look for brainstem signs: cranial nerve signs ± long tract signs, divergent squint, pupillary and doll's eye reflex loss
Supratentorial (structural lesion)	Asymmetrical long tract signs without brain stem signs (may be false localizing III, IV, or VI if mass effect or aneurysm), focal seizures, conjugate eye deviation
Toxic-metabolic	Confusion and drowsiness with few motor signs
	Motor signs symmetrical
	Pupillary responses preserved
	Myoclonus, asterixis (flap), tremulousness, and seizures common
	Acid–base imbalance
Psychogenic	Eyes tight shut
	Pupils reactive
	Doll's eye and caloric reflexes preserved
	Motor tone normal or inconsistent resistance to movement
	Reflexes normal
	EEG shows wakefulness

Diagnosing stroke

You need a careful history. If the patient is unconscious, unable to communicate (e.g. aphasic), or confused, that is no excuse—ask someone else. If an informant is not immediately present, use the telephone. There may be old hospital case notes available, paper or electronic. Look at them, and briefly summarize useful information.

You need to know:
- What happened, and what the current symptoms are.
- The time of onset, and time-course of progression.
- If it has happened before (previous stroke, TIA).
- Past medical and drug history (prescription, over the counter and illicit—nasal decongestants, amphetamines, and cocaine can cause strokes).
- Vascular risk factors.
- Previous functional, occupational, and cognitive ability (including driving).
- Information useful for rehabilitation and discharge planning—type of accommodation, cohabitation (and the health of an often-elderly cohabitee), family, and other domestic support.
- Family history of stroke or thrombotic disease (occasionally gives a diagnostic clue, may also reveal previous knowledge, experiences or expectations).

Some of this can be collected later on, if necessary. But admission is a good opportunity to be thorough.

History taking (and examination) is an inductive process. Use the information you gather to formulate hypotheses about what is going on, which you test with new questions. You want evidence that this is a stroke, and to rule in or rule out other diagnoses. You also want to put the new pathology in context by documenting comorbid conditions, and their disabling consequences.

Examination

General

A thorough general examination is required, because:

- The patient may be very ill, and require securing of the airway, breathing, and circulation before an adequate assessment can be made.
- The possibility of a condition mimicking or causing stroke (AF, malignancy, endocarditis).
- The importance of comorbidity in a generally elderly population.

The cardiovascular system is examined routinely, but the mental state and musculoskeletal systems, in particular, are often overlooked. An admissions ward or Emergency Department is not always the best place to examine these properly.

Initially test cognition using simple orientation (person, place, and time) and short-term memory, or the 10-point Abbreviated Mental Test (AMT, 📖 Appendix 1, p.324). Later on, use the 30-point Folstein Mini-Mental State Examination (MMSE, 📖 Appendix 2, p.324).

Blood pressure (BP) may be raised (or very raised), but the ward record over the next hours, days, and weeks will give a better picture of 'usual' BP. The pulse may be slowed in raised intracranial pressure, or irregular in AF. There may be periodic (Cheyne–Stokes) respiration, or evidence of chest infection. Routinely record pulse oximetry.

Neurological examination

Is directed at:

- Identifying features which require special precautions (e.g. coma, dysphagia).
- Defining a clinical stroke syndrome (localizing the lesion).
- Quantifying neurological impairments as a baseline for subsequent improvements or deteriorations.
- Raising suspicion of alternative, non-stroke, diagnoses.

The routine examination—cranial nerves, limb tone, power, reflexes, co-ordination, and sensation—should be followed, but some aspects need emphasizing, and others need adapting. You cannot examine co-ordination in a paralysed limb, or assess subtle parietal lobe signs in a drowsy patient.

- At minimum in an *unconscious, uncomprehending, or uncooperative patient*, and with a little ingenuity, you can record eye movements, facial weakness, limb tone, and gross power, and usually reflexes.
- *Level of consciousness*: this is important for prognosis and immediate nursing care. Use the Glasgow Coma Scale (GCS) (📖 Appendix 3, p.325). Describe the response if you cannot remember the numbers. There is a clear problem in underestimating level of consciousness in aphasia, but it is familiar and well-understood. The 'AVPU' system (Alert, rousable to Voice, rousable to Pain, Unconscious) is a valid alternative.
- Check for a *stiff neck*, and for evidence of *head trauma*.
- Examine the *fundi* for papilloedema, retinopathy, or subhyaloid haemorrhage.

- If unconscious:
  - Check *brainstem function*—pupillary reaction to light, doll's eye movements, corneal reflexes, gag reflex.
  - The *caloric reflex* is sometimes useful. Can be used after cervical spine trauma:
    - check the tympanic membrane is intact and there is no wax, then inject 20mL of ice cold water into the ear canal. Conjugate eye movement towards stimulated ear indicates that the midbrain/pons is intact.
    - absent or dysconjugate response implies brainstem damage at the level of the pons or sedative drug intoxication.
  - Loss of *pupillary reaction to light* implies a midbrain lesion.
  - Pontine lesions can cause small but reactive pupils.
  - Dysconjugate gaze indicates a palsy of cranial nerves III, IV, or VI (nuclei in the midbrain and pons) or their connections (medial longitudinal fasciculus), a false localizing sign in raised intracranial pressure, a mimic such as myasthenia gravis, or a congenital squint.
  - Conjugate deviation of the eyes suggests either a frontal lobe infarct on the same side as the direction of gaze, an irritative lesion (tumour, haemorrhage) of the opposite frontal lobe, or a pontine lesion in the opposite lateral gaze centre.
  - No eye movement at all indicates a pontine lesion, or a mimic such as Guillain–Barré syndrome.
- Check the *visual fields*, upper and lower quadrants. Also, if possible, test for *visual inattention* (visual extinction—inability to perceive a stimulus when a simultaneous stimulus is presented to the other visual field, in the absence of a visual field defect). Wiggling fingers are sufficient for the purpose, rather than coloured pin heads.
- Record *speech* impairment: dysarthria, receptive aphasia, expressive aphasia. Test receptive ability (understanding, following commands) first using instructions with a non-verbal response (e.g. 'close your eyes', 'touch your left ear'). If there is reasonable understanding, then test for expressive aphasia (spontaneous speech, naming, sequences such as counting, yes/no responses).
- Test *swallowing*—with the patient sitting up, give small sips (or spoonfuls) of water, and, from behind, feel for prompt laryngeal elevation. Observe for delay, aspiration (choking or coughing), or 'wetness' of the voice. Tap water is more or less sterile. You produce a litre of saliva a day, which is far from sterile. Many hospitals have nurse-delivered swallow testing protocols, which should be used.
- The presence or absence of the gag reflex tells you nothing about the safety of swallowing.
- Examine *motor function*:
  - Examine power in the face, arm, and leg.
  - 'Pronator drift' is a good test for subtle deficits—the downward drifting and pronation of hands held stretched out horizontally in front, with palms upwards and eyes closed (Fig. 1.1).
  - Weakness follows a 'pyramidal distribution'. Shoulder abduction, elbow extension, and wrist dorsiflexion will be weaker than corresponding flexor functions, and hip and knee flexion and foot dorsiflexion will be weaker than extensor functions.

- Carefully test limb *tone* and *reflexes*, especially in mild cases. If the reflexes are very brisk, try the pectoral jerks, and Hoffman's reflex (thumb flexion when the terminal phalanx of the middle finger is flexed under tension then suddenly released with a 'flick'), where asymmetry may be easier to detect (Fig. 1.2).
- Test *coordination*, and *gait* if possible. If not, assess head and trunk control (sitting balance).
- Test *sensation*:
  - There may be spinothalamic sensory loss (temperature, pin prick/pain).
  - More useful are some 'cortical sensory modalities', often as part of a search for 'cortical involvement' when identifying a stroke syndrome:
    ○ stereognosis (identifying objects in the hand).
    ○ graphaesthesia (identifying numbers traced on the hand).
  - Test for sensory inattention (similar to visual inattention, using touch instead of visual stimuli).
- If possible, test for other cortical or parietal functions, including:
  - Neglect (Albert's test/line cancellation, drawing a clock face, or double-headed daisy)
  - Apraxia (drawing tasks—intersecting pentagons, five-pointed star)
  - Sometimes specific dyscalculia (sums), dyslexia (reading), or dysgraphia (writing)
  - Body image and proprioception can be assessed using the 'thumb-finding test' (affected arm supported in front, eyes closed, the patient is asked to find their thumb with their unaffected hand).

Some of these tests can wait for a few days. However, signs may resolve rapidly.

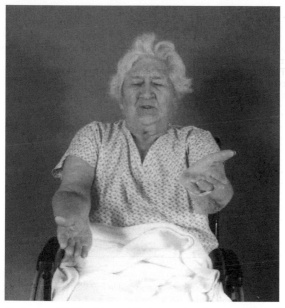

Fig. 1.1 Pronator drift. The right arm drifts downwards and pronates when held out in front with eyes shut.

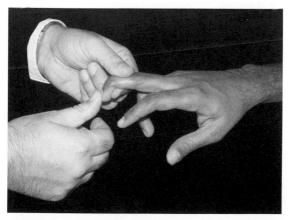

Fig. 1.2 Hoffman's reflex. After flexing and suddenly releasing the terminal phalanx, the thumb flexes if the reflex is positive.

Investigations

- First check blood glucose with a portable glucometer (e.g. BM stick).
- Get a CT head scan (or MRI) as soon as possible after admission, unless the diagnosis is certain and the patient is moribund (which will be rare). The scan is to diagnose or exclude bleeds and stroke mimics rather than to confirm infarction.
- CT scan should be urgent if thrombolysis is possible, or if there is suspicion of:
  - Trauma.
  - Cerebellar haematoma.
  - Subarachnoid haemorrhage.
  - Raised intracranial pressure.
  - If level of consciousness is deteriorating or fluctuating.
  - There is undiagnosed coma.
  - If the patient is on anticoagulants, or needs anticoagulation (or antithrombotics, if a bleed is suspected).
  - Known bleeding disorder.
- MRI is better at diagnosing lacunar and posterior fossa infarcts. Diffusion-weighted imaging (DWI) becomes positive after about 30min of ischaemia and remains so for up to 2 weeks, and is the most sensitive way of diagnosing (and excluding) an acute infarct.
- Half of TIAs have positive DWI. If there is doubt about diagnosis or vascular territory then this is the investigation of choice in TIA. But you cannot completely rule out short-duration cerebral ischaemia with MRI.
- Blood count, electrolytes, including calcium, glucose, renal, liver, and thyroid function, erythrocyte sedimentation rate (ESR), or C-reactive protein and urinalysis should be done routinely. Check coagulation if on anticoagulants, or if proposing them, or if the scan shows a bleed. Measure cholesterol, if within 2 days of the stroke.
- Electrocardiogram (ECG) in everyone.
- Ideally get an echocardiogram in potentially embolic (partial anterior and posterior circulation) strokes. But the call for echocardiography is high and the diagnostic yield low. Local services may limit this to cases where there is other clinical or ECG evidence of heart disease. Younger patients with no other apparent cause for stroke should have transoesophageal or transthoracic echocardiography with bubble contrast to look for patent foramen ovale (PFO, Box 1.1).
- You are unlikely to get a technically decent chest X-ray. In any case you are more likely to diagnose malignancy from the CT head scan than the chest X-ray. Don't request routinely unless there are specific chest problems or signs you want to investigate (e.g. unexplained fever, or presumed aspiration pneumonia).
- Carotid duplex scan if anterior circulation stroke resulting in no more than minor disability, and the patient would be willing to undergo carotid endarterectomy. Also detects about half of carotid dissections.

- CT or magnetic resonance angiography (MRA)—to diagnose dissection, as a prelude to carotid endarterectomy, or to investigate intracranial bleeding (from an aneurysm or AVM) when neurosurgery is contemplated.
- Ambulatory ECG (24-h tape) is rarely necessary. Paroxysmal AF (that would not have been detected otherwise) can be found on 24-h ECG monitoring in about 5% of patients who have had a stroke. Consider it where the aetiology remains unclear, and cardiac embolism is suspected (cortical lesions in different vascular territories).
- Additional tests may be required in younger stroke patients (aged <50 years). See 📖 Stroke in younger adults, p.24.
- Following haemorrhage, angiography should be performed in patients who:
  - Are under 50, or
  - Have lobar or unusual pattern, suggesting possibility of an underlying aneurysm, AVM, or tumour on CT or MRI.

An interval MRI scan at 6–12 weeks (or longer, when the blood has fully resorbed and the oedema settled) may be required to exclude an underlying lesion. Routinely discuss these cases with a neuroradiologist.

Box 1.1 Patent foramen ovale (PFO) and cryptogenic stroke

- 227 patients with cryptogenic cerebral infarction (i.e. in whom a mechanism could not be determined), were compared with 276 where a cause was found, in a case–control study. Prevalence of PFO and atrial septal aneurysm were determined by transoesophageal echocardiography.
- Odds ratios for stroke in the presence of a PFO were:
  - 4.7 (95% CI 1.9–11.7) for those ≤55 years (44% vs 14%).
  - 2.9 (95% CI 1.7–5.0) for those ≥55 years (28% vs 12%).
- Odds ratios for stroke in the presence of a PFO with atrial septal aneurysm were:
  - 7.4 (95% CI 1.01–327) for those ≤55 years (13% vs 2%).
  - 3.9 (95% CI 1.8–8.5) for those ≥55 years (15% vs 4%).
- Associations were independent of other stroke risk factors.
- Results suggest (by calculating population attributable risk fraction) that a third of cryptogenic stroke in those ≤55, and a 20% in those >55 years, could be due to paradoxical embolism.

NEJM 2007; **357**:2262–8.

Clinical subtypes

Stroke is a mixed bag of pathologies. These include intracerebral and subarachnoid bleeding, and infarction. Infarction divides between large vessel disease, small end-artery (lacunar) disease, cardioembolism, and rare causes such as venous infarction, vasculitis, and infective endocarditis.

Primary intracerebral haemorrhage

Bleeds occur in the cerebral lobes, basal ganglia, thalamus, brain stem (especially pons), and cerebellum. Cytotoxic and vasogenic oedema forms around them over the next 2–4 days.

Acute bleeds have some characteristic features:
- Apoplectic onset (sudden loss of consciousness).
- Headache.
- Vomiting.
- Stiff neck.

Unfortunately, these, and various scoring systems derived from combinations of them (such as the Guy's diagnostic and Siriraj scores), are insufficiently accurate for clinical use. Small bleeds, and bleeds seen very early (e.g. within 3h of onset), are clinically indistinguishable from infarcts.

An early CT scan is required to make the diagnosis. The request should be urgent where subarachnoid haemorrhage is suspected (to initiate medical management, and part of the work-up to exclude meningitis), or if the patient is on anticoagulants (early reversal may limit growth of the haematoma). Haematomas absorb over 10–30 days. Leave the scan longer than a week, and a small bleed may have resolved on CT (although MRI can still detect haemoglobin breakdown products).

Haematomas tend to enlarge over the first few hours after onset (25% enlarge in the first hour, 40% over the first day), especially when aspirin or anticoagulants have been taken. Growth of the haematoma is associated with early neurological deterioration.

Table 1.4 Pathology of intracerebral haemorrhage

Type	Features
Charcot–Bouchard microaneurysms	Lipohyalinosis, often associated with hypertension, causes weakness of the walls of small perforating arteries, usually to the basal ganglia, thalamus, or pons
Amyloid angiopathy	Commonest cause of lobar haemorrhage in the over 60s. Affects small arteries particularly in the meninges and superficial cortex. Arteries are weakened by fibrinoid degeneration, amyloid deposition, segmental dilatation, and microaneurysm formation. Affects men and women equally, especially those with dementia. Resulting haematoma is usually superficial and lobar. Often recur
Berry aneurysms	Comprise majority of intracranial aneurysms. Thin-walled saccular dilatation of the arteries, may be multiloculated if large. Probably acquired rather than congenital. Most are small. Found in 2–5% of autopsies. Associated with age, hypertension, and atheroma. Found at distal end of the arteries, mainly at circle of Willis—carotid tree 75%; basilar tree 10%; both 15%. Rupture causes subarachnoid haemorrhage, but may extend into the brain substance or ventricles
Fusiform aneurysms	Found on atheromatous large arteries (internal carotid, basilar) in elderly people, due to replacement of the muscular layer by fibrous tissue. A common site is the supraclinoid segment of the internal carotid artery. A complication is compression of structures in the cavernous sinus wall
Arteriovenous malformations	Consist of a mass of enlarged and tortuous vessels. Supplied by one or more large arteries. Drained by one or more large veins. They are congenital and may run in families. Present with recurrent headaches, epilepsy, subarachnoid or intracerebral haemorrhages. Commonest site is on the middle cerebral artery
Secondary haemorrhage	Due to anticoagulant therapy, thrombolytic therapy (e.g. for heart attack), haemorrhagic disease, bleeding into tumours or mycotic aneurysms, or haemorrhagic transformation of an infarct

Infarcts

Pathological mechanisms

A good level of diagnostic acumen and clinical suspicion is needed to detect rare but treatable causes of infarction such as infective endocarditis (peripheral stigmata, new murmurs, raised inflammatory markers, positive blood cultures), cerebral vasculitis, thrombophilia, or venous infarction.

Once these have been excluded, we are left with the majority of patients, who have cerebral infarction due to arterial thrombosis or embolism.

If we are to direct further investigation and management logically, ideally we need to know more than just that a stroke has occurred. Table 1.5 gives some different pathological mechanisms. Sometimes we can work out exactly why the stroke occurred. In practice, however, up to 40% of causes remain undetermined despite comprehensive work-up.

Table 1.5 Pathology of cerebral infarction

Type	Features
Cardiac emboli	About 20% of ischaemic strokes. Half of cases are due to AF; other causes include mitral stenosis and prosthetic valves, mural thrombus after myocardial infarction (MI), left ventricular aneurysm, dilated cardiomyopathy, atrial myxoma, patent foramen ovale with paradoxical embolism of venous thrombi. Typically results in peripherally-located, wedge-shaped infarcts, often becoming haemorrhagic. Can involve multiple arterial distributions
Large vessel disease	Atherosclerosis of aorta, common carotid, and internal carotid artery. Stenosis, plaque rupture, and ulceration, platelet aggregation, and red cell thrombus formation, may cause occlusion or provide a source of emboli. Internal carotid artery clot may propagate into the middle cerebral artery. Otherwise perfusion is dependent on collaterals from the Circle of Willis
Small vessel (lacunar) disease	Lipohyalinosis or microatheroma of small end arteries, associated with hypertension, diabetes mellitus, or hyperlipidaemia
Arterial dissection (carotid or vertebral)	About 5% of ischaemic stroke <65 years of age, sometimes following trauma or unusual neck movements. May have pain in the neck or face, and an ipsilateral Horner's syndrome
Arterial boundary-zone ('watershed') infarction	May complicate hypotension or cardiac arrest. Damage is variable. Usually bilateral, often parieto-occipital (between MCA and PCA territories), causing cortical blindness, visual disorientation, amnesia, agnosia. The ACA-MCA boundary can be compromised due to unilateral ICA stenosis or occlusion, causing predominant leg weakness or sensory loss, with facial sparing. Other patterns are possible, including cortical sensory loss, aphasia, hemianopia, motor weakness
Post-subarachnoid haemorrhage	Infarction occurs within 4–12 days in 25% of patients with subarachnoid haemorrhage, due to arterial spasm
Rare causes	Infective endocarditis, vasculitis (e.g. giant cell arteritis, SLE), subclavian steal, hyperviscosity, and prothrombotic conditions, postpartum, iatrogenic causes (internal jugular cannulation, cerebral angiography, or cardiac catheterization)

Oxfordshire Community Stroke Project classification (Table 1.6)

The OCSP anatomical classification localizes stroke lesions on clinical grounds, and indicates likely pathology and prognosis.

- Posterior circulation infarcts (POCIs) are mostly thrombotic (80%), the rest embolic (20%).
- Lacunar infarcts (LACIs) are due to thrombotic occlusions of small, deep, end-arteries.
- Partial anterior circulation infarcts (PACIs) are predominantly embolic
- Total anterior circulation infarcts (TACIs) split between embolic (2/3) and in situ thrombosis (1/3).

Clinical stroke type agrees well with anatomical localization on CT scan (although lacunar and partial anterior circulation strokes are least reliably distinguished). Strictly the scheme applies only to infarcts, but in practice is sometimes applied to bleeds as well, the 'I' for infarct becoming 'S' for stroke or syndrome (TACS, PACS, etc.).

Table 1.6 Oxfordshire Community Stroke Project Stroke classification

Type	Features
Posterior circulation infarct (POCI)	Cranial nerve deficit with contralateral hemiparesis or sensory deficit, or bilateral stroke, or disorders of conjugate eye movement, or isolated cerebellar stroke, or isolated homonymous hemianopia
Lacunar infarcts (LACI)	Pure motor or pure sensory deficit affecting 2 out of 3 of face, arm, and leg, or sensorimotor stroke (basal ganglia and internal capsule), or ataxic hemiparesis (cerebellar-type ataxia with ipsilateral pyramidal signs—internal capsule or pons); or dysarthria plus clumsy hand, or acute onset movement disorders (hemichorea, hemiballismus—basal ganglia)
Total anterior circulation infarct (TACI)	1. New higher cerebral function dysfunction: aphasia/dyscalculia/apraxia/neglect/visuospatial problems plus 2. Homonymous visual field defect, plus 3. Hemimotor and/or sensory deficit of at least 2 areas of face, arm, and leg motor and sensory deficit. In the presence of impaired consciousness, higher cerebral function and visual fields deficits are assumed
Partial anterior circulation infarct (PACI)	2 of the 3 components of TACI, or isolated aphasia or other cortical dysfunction, or motor/sensory loss more limited than for a LACI

Data from *Lancet* 1991; **337**:1521–6.

Brainstem strokes

Brainstem strokes can be missed, but are also overdiagnosed, because the individual elements are non-specific (like diplopia or vertigo), meaning that they can be caused by a number of different pathologies. It is the specific combination of neurological signs and symptoms that indicate the focal nature of the lesion. Small pontine infarcts can cause lacunar syndromes. However, the classical pattern for a brainstem stroke is an ipsilateral cranial nerve palsy with a contralateral hemiparesis. Some of the specific patterns are listed in Table 1.7.

Basilar artery occlusion

Complete occlusion has a mortality of 80%, but partial or intermittent occlusion is also possible. The clinical course is can be stuttering and progressive, over days or weeks. Causes can be *in situ* thrombosis, embolism, and vertebral artery dissection.

Symptoms and signs are variable, depending on the level of the occlusion (i.e. any of the posterior circulation strokes), and the state of collateral flow. Symptoms include:

- Oculomotor and limb weakness.
- Headache.
- Vertigo.
- Drowsiness or coma.
- Dysarthria.

Up to 70% have hemiparesis or quadriparesis. 40% have pupillary abnormalities, oculomotor signs (III, VI, internuclear ophthalmoplegia, conjugate gaze defects), and bulbar palsy (facial weakness, dysphonia, dysarthria, dysphagia).

'Top of the basilar syndrome' is usually due to an embolus. Presents with abnormal conscious level, visual symptoms (hallucinations, cortical blindness), abnormal eye movements (usually of vertical gaze), third nerve palsy and pupillary abnormalities, and abnormal motor movements or posturing.

Coma with oculomotor abnormalities and quadriplegia indicates pontine damage due to midbasilar occlusion.

'Locked-in' syndrome comprises complete paralysis apart from blinking and vertical eye movements. The patient is aware and alert (i.e. can potentially respond purposefully to external stimuli). Caused by proximal basilar occlusion.

MRI and MRA are the investigations of choice.

Table 1.7 Brainstem strokes

Level		Neurological signs by side		Eponym
		Ipsilateral	Contralateral	
Midbrain	Rostral	Paralysis of upward (± downward) conjugate gaze, convergence, absent light reflex		Parinaud
	Dorsolateral	Horner's ± cerebellar	Total sensory loss	
	Paramedian	III	Cerebellar ataxia, tremor, (+ hemiparesis, hemisensory)	Claude (Benedikt)
	Basal	III	Hemiplegia	Weber
Pons	Dorsolateral	Horner's, cerebellar, ± VII (sensory), ± gaze palsy	Spinothalamic sensory loss	
	Paramedian	VI, gaze palsy	± Spinothalamic sensory loss	
	Basal	VI, LMN VII	Hemiplegia ± UMN VII	Millard–Gubler
	Basal	LMN VII, gaze palsy towards lesion	Hemiplegia	Foville
	Bilateral ventral	Locked-in syndrome		
Medulla	Lateral	Horner's, facial spinothalamic loss (pain, temperature), cerebellar ataxia, LMN VII,VIII (vertigo, vomiting), IX, X (dysphagia)	Corporal spinothalamic sensory loss	Wallenberg
	Central	XII	Hemiplegia, dorsal column sensory loss	

Stroke in younger adults

10% of strokes occur in people <50 years of age.

Be on the alert for something unusual. There is little fundamentally different about stroke in younger people. You still need to arrive at an explanation for what has happened, and many of the rarer causes of stroke also arise in older adults. About 30% of strokes in younger adults remain unexplained despite investigation.

Atherosclerotic vascular disease does occur in adults <50 years, but is relatively less common. Bleeds, cardiogenic stroke, and stroke mimics are all proportionately more common.

Particular diagnoses to consider are:
- Arterial dissection.
- Paradoxical embolism via a PFO.
- Substance abuse.
- Bleeding disorders and prothrombotic states.
- Vasculitis.
- Fabry's disease or other genetic disorders.

Table 1.8 Additional tests in younger patients

Condition	Test	Comments
Arterial dissection	Neck MRI, MRA, CTA, angiography	High index of suspicion in patients <50 years, otherwise look out for clinical clues
Substance abuse	History, blood, and urine toxicology	Cocaine, amphetamine and heroin. Cause vasospasm, hypertension or vasculitis. Watch for endocarditis
Clotting disorders		
Sickle cell disease	Hb electrophoresis	Afro-Caribbean people
Thrombophilia	Protein S and C deficiencies, antithrombin III, Factor V Leiden/ PC resistance, prothrombin 20210A	Usually cause venous thromboses, but sometimes arterial disease, or cause paradoxical embolism
Antiphospholipid syndrome	Persistent (over 6 weeks) anti-cardiolipin antibody, or lupus anticoagulant, with thrombosis, foetal loss, thrombocytopaenia	May be primary or secondary (connective tissue disorders, infections, drugs). Most commonly venous thrombosis, but also cerebral arteries. 20% of thromboses are cerebral—arterial or venous. Recurrence common (9% per year)
Hyperhomocysteinaemia	Homocysteine (random or post-methionine load)	Treatment uncertain; folic acid, B_{12} and pyridoxine reduce homocysteine level but not ri

Table 1.8 *(Contd.)*

Condition	Test	Comments
Oestrogens	History (post-partum, combined oral contraceptive, HRT)	May also cause venous sinus thrombosis
Waldenstrom's macroglobulinaemia	ESR, protein electrophoresis, plasma viscosity	More often hyperviscosity syndrome (drowsy, headache, ataxia, diplopia, visual blurring, dysarthria)
Malignancy	History, blood tests, imaging	Especially GI, breast and gynaecological. Warfarin may not control thrombosis risk
Bleeding disorders	FBC, PT/INR, APTT, FDP	Anticoagulants, thrombolytics, leukaemia, platelet disorders, DIC, haemophilia
Vasculitis	Clinical features (headache, weight loss, fever, malaise, jaw claudication, scalp tenderness, polymyalgia, rash, joint or renal problems, anaemia); ESR; ds-DNA; ANCA; temporal artery, skin, renal or brain biopsy; MRI	Can be primary, otherwise connective tissue disorders, Sjögren's, Behçet's, sarcoid. Diagnosis may be known. MRI shows meningeal inflammation and areas of patchy infarction or haemorrhage. Angiography may be helpful but is non-specific. Also causes bleeds
PFO with paradoxical embolism	Bubble contrast echocardiography with Valsalva manoeuvre	Low threshold for transoesophageal or bubble contrast echo if no likely non-cardiac source, but difficult to establish causality
Fabry's disease	Alpha-galactosidase A activity and genetic analysis	X-linked inheritance, males predominate. Causes early cerebral vasculopathy, ischaemic strokes, and TIAs. Also cardiac, renal, skin, eye, gut, and peripheral nerve involvement, with neuropathic pain a common presentation
Cerebral autosomal dominant arteriopathy with subcortical infarcts and leukoencephalopathy (CADASIL)	MRI	Hereditary small vessel arteriopathy. Presents in middle age. Migraine, recurrent lacunar strokes, and later dementia
Mitochondrial encephalomyopathy with lactic acidosis and stroke-like episodes (MELAS)	MRI, plasma and CSF lactate, mitochondrial DNA analysis (mutation A3243G)	Typically produces strokes in non-arterial distributions. Often occipital lobe strokes at young age (children, adults <40 years), fits, multiple other problems

Carotid and vertebral arterial dissection

The arterial wall splits, blood enters the intima, resulting in an intramural haematoma, and a true and a false lumen. Ischaemic stroke results from:
- Embolism from thrombus within the true lumen, or
- Occlusion of the true lumen by the dissection or thrombus.

Spontaneous arterial dissection occurs in atheroma, cystic medial necrosis, fibromuscular dysplasia, Ehlers–Danlos and Marfan's syndromes. Intracranial (especially vertebrobasilar) dissection can cause subarachnoid haemorrhage.

Features include:
- History of neck trauma (including rotation, hyperextension, and penetrating injuries), but this is absent in most.
- Pain in one of the following areas:
  - Face.
  - Around the eye.
  - Neck (ipsilateral to carotid dissection).
  - Unusual unilateral headache.
  - Occiput and back of the neck (vertebral dissection).
- May have no neurological signs.
- 10–20% experience TIA.
- Ipsilateral Horner's syndrome due to damage to the sympathetic fibres around the internal carotid artery (20%).
- Ipsilateral lower cranial nerve palsies (12%, particularly hypoglossal, due to pressure from the internal carotid wall at the base of the skull).
- Contralateral motor, visual, or higher cortical function deficits.
- Note that the combination of ipsilateral cranial nerve and contralateral pyramidal lesions mimics brainstem strokes.
- The pain and Horner's syndrome may precede stroke by a few days to 4 weeks.
- Consider skin and joint hyperextensibility, abnormal scars, and retinal abnormalities.

Investigation
- The definitive investigation is cerebral angiography, usually MRA or CT angiography (CTA), but may also be seen on carotid duplex scanning and neck MRI (Fig. 1.3, the intramural haematoma is visible as a 'crescent sign' in the carotid wall in the neck on T2 imaging; see Fig. 1.3c).
- If the carotid is completely occluded by the dissection, imaging is non-specific.
- Imaging must be done within days of symptom onset, because the dissection may resolve spontaneously (30% within 8 days, 60–80% within 3 months).

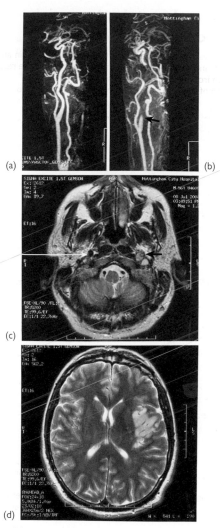

Fig. 1.3 Carotid dissection. a) MR angiogram, normal right carotid bifurcation.
b) MR angiogram showing tapering occlusion of left internal carotid artery (arrow).
c) T2-weighted MRI showing mural haematoma in left internal carotid artery (crescent sign, thick arrow). Note normal flow void of right internal carotid artery (thin arrow).
d) T2-weighted MRI showing small infarct in left insular cortex. The patient presented with aphasia and persisting left facial pain.

Leukoaraiosis

Leukoaraiosis is a term describing subcortical white matter changes seen as hyperintensities on T2-weighted MRI, and as patchy hypodensities on CT. It is thought to represent chronic small vessel white matter ischaemic change, although the precise explanation of how it arises is uncertain.

Age, hypertension, smoking, diabetes, carotid atheroma, and heart disease are all risk factors. The appearance is associated (albeit inconsistently) with gait disturbance and cognitive impairment (especially attention, processing speed, and executive function, but also other aspects of vascular dementia). It is associated with increased risk of both cerebral infarction and haemorrhage. Whether the appearance warrants vascular prevention drugs is uncertain, but many people with it will justify this on primary prevention grounds in any case.

Summary

1. Stroke is a clinical syndrome—*a rapidly developing episode of focal or global neurological dysfunction, lasting >24h or leading to death, and of presumed vascular origin.*

2. Diagnosis can be difficult. The deficit may progress over 24h or more, the presentation may be atypical, and some alternative diagnoses are difficult to make.

3. At least 10% of presumed strokes reaching hospital will have another diagnosis.

4. The neurological deficits depend on where the stroke is and how big it is. Hence, it is quite variable, but a number of distinct patterns can be identified.

5. The OCSP clinical classification gives useful information about the extent of neurological deficit, aetiology, prognosis, and recurrence rates.

6. An attempt should be made at elucidating the pathology underlying the stroke—unless the patient is clearly moribund and no active intervention is contemplated. Most important are the clinical stroke subtype, CT or MRI scans, blood glucose, electrolytes, ECG, and inflammatory markers.

7. If there is pain or neck trauma, or in younger patients, consider arterial dissection. In younger patients also consider the possibility of substance abuse.

Chapter 2

What to do in the first few days

How health services help

Health care has seven main functions (Table 2.1). Tasks are shared between doctors, nurses, and other health professionals.

The first day

The first task on seeing any patient is to make a rapid evaluation of immediate resuscitation needs, and act if necessary. Assess:
- Airway.
- Breathing.
- Circulation.

Ask urgently about the time of onset, and consider if it is possible to deliver thrombolysis within 4.5h of onset? If it is:
- Make sure family members or informants remain available.
- Alert the CT department of an immediate need for a scan.
- Call for help: a unit offering thrombolysis will have a protocol to ensure its rapid and safe delivery. It will require more than one person. Follow the guidelines as shown on ⊞ Thrombolysis, p.38, Appendices 5 and 6.
- Insert a venous cannula and take blood.
- If you need to move the patient to another hospital for possible thrombolysis, request emergency transport, and immediately confirm your plan with a senior clinical decision maker so that time is not lost.

Otherwise, tasks for the first day include:
- Making, confirming, or refuting the diagnosis.
- Documenting comorbid conditions or complications.
- Understanding the immediate context of the disease, including its severity and resulting disabilities, other complicating medical factors, and sufficient background social information to allow decisions on the need for admission to hospital, or the scope for early discharge.
- Ordering initial investigations.
- Initial specific medical management.
- Making risk assessments for pressure areas, moving and handling, nutrition, bed rails, and falls.
- Instigating plans for maintaining oxygenation, relief of pressure areas, feeding and hydration, and bladder and bowel management.
- Physiological monitoring.
- Management of immediate complications and comorbid conditions.
- Making initial referrals to rehabilitation therapists.
- Communicating the diagnosis and plans to patients, their relatives, and medical and nursing colleagues.

Pre-written care pathways can help ensure that assessments and interventions are systematic, comprehensive, and made at the right time (⊞ Appendix 4, p.326).

Table 2.1 Seven functions of health care

Function	Example in stroke care
Prevention of disease, or complications of disease	Manipulation of vascular risk factors; aspirin or anticoagulants in vascular disease; prevention of pressure sores, dehydration, malnutrition, aspiration pneumonia, venous thrombosis, joint contractures, institutionalization
Cure of disease, or complications of disease	Thrombolysis in acute stroke; antibiotics for infections; healing of pressure sores; feeding in malnutrition; antidepressants for biological depression (?)
Prolonging life, deferring death	Organized multidisciplinary stroke care; antibiotics for pneumonia; aspirin, statins, and antihypertensive drugs as secondary prevention
Palliation of unpleasant symptoms	Analgesia for pain; mouth care if nil by mouth; management of anxiety and depression; drugs for spasticity; management of incontinence; many treatments of comorbid conditions
Maximize physical and social function (rehabilitation)	Physiotherapy, occupational therapy, rehabilitation nursing, speech therapy, goal setting, discharge planning, environmental changes
Information	Explanation of diagnosis and its effects; advising on secondary prevention; giving prognosis
Support for families and other carers	Reassurance; training in care-giving; concern, empathy and sympathy; positive outlook; realistic planning

Whether and where to admit?

The great majority of stroke patients should be admitted to hospital. Do so unless:

- Functional impairment is minimal (but look carefully: subtle executive function and visuospatial problems are easy to miss, and may not be revealed without an assessment by an occupational therapist).
- The patient can be seen in an appropriate clinic and investigated the same day (or within a few days). The clinic should be able to confirm the diagnosis and identify residual disabilities and secondary prevention needs. Such clinics should have immediate access to CT or MRI and carotid duplex scanning (see 📖 Neurovascular or TIA clinics, p.274).
- The patient has severe pre-existing chronic disabilities, often a nursing home resident. Admission may have little to offer in terms of nursing care, sensible investigation, or treatment. In experienced hands, this can represent good, humane, and appropriate care. Such a decision is not easy to make, and may require specialist consultation to support it. If handled poorly, decisions not to admit can be discriminatory, or lead to self-fulfilling prophesies (outcome is poor not because it was inevitable, but because potentially useful treatments were not given).

The rationale for hospital admission is:

- Potentially curative treatments (thrombolysis) may be given, and haemorrhages or stroke mimics diagnosed that may require urgent treatment.
- Patients value admission. They and their families are suddenly met with frightening or bewildering symptoms (like hemiparesis and aphasia), need reassurance that they are being cared for, and have the support of people who have seen it before, know what they are doing, and can offer the best chances of return to normal abilities.
- Coordinated, specialist, inpatient stroke care prevents unnecessary deaths, disability, and dependency (compared with care on general medical wards), suggesting that some aspects of hospital care are important in determining outcomes.
- A controlled trial in the 1980s found that a home-based care team increased admission rates, probably by uncovering previously unmet needs.
- A randomized trial comparing admission to a stroke unit; home-based, multi-disciplinary specialist care; and a peripatetic team who supported management on general medical wards found decisively in favour of the stroke unit (Box 2.1).

Admission should be directly to a specialist acute stroke unit. The FAST test (Box 2.2) applied by paramedics or ambulance staff is sufficiently accurate for this purpose.

Direct admission minimizes delays when thrombolysis is planned, allows immediate expertise in diagnosis, monitoring, and intervention; prevention, detection, and management of early complications; and assessment for rehabilitation needs and early hospital discharge.

Box 2.1 Orpington models of care trial

- 467 acute patients within 72h of stroke, with persisting disability, but who were fit enough to consider home management, were randomized between stroke unit care, specialist home care supported by a stroke physician, or general ward care supported by a mobile stroke team (see 🕮 Box 3.5, p.93).
- 34% of the domiciliary group were subsequently admitted to the hospital stroke unit.
- Mortality or institutionalization at 1 year was 14% for the stroke unit, 24% for home care (including those transferred to the stroke unit), and 30% for supported general ward care. The main reduction was in mortality.
- Proportions alive without severe disability at 1 year were 85% (in-patient stroke unit), 71% (specialized home care), and 66% (general medical ward with mobile stroke team).

Lancet 2000; **356**:894–9.

Box 2.2 FAST: the Face, Arm, and Speech Test

- A quick and easy test for possible stroke.
- FACE—ask patient to smile. Do both sides of the face move the same?
- ARM—ask patient to lift both arms out in front of them and hold them there. Is one side weaker than the other?
- SPEECH—in simple conversation (How are you? What happened?) is speech slurred, hesitant, unintelligible, or completely absent?

If any of these is abnormal, the test is positive, and there is a strong possibility of a stroke. Sensitivity and specificity are both about 80%. That means about 80% of all patients with stroke are 'FAST positive', and about 80% of patients who are 'FAST positive' have had a stroke. Posterior circulation strokes are underdiagnosed.

Management of coma

- You may admit patients who are unconscious, with a working diagnosis of stroke. Initially the diagnosis is uncertain.
- If the diagnosis is stroke, the outlook is poor but not hopeless. In addition, toxic, metabolic, or other comorbidity may be complicating the picture.
- The aim is to provide resuscitation and supportive treatment while a diagnosis is made, and allowing definitive management to be instituted.
- If maintaining the airway is at risk, consult an anaesthetist or intensivist urgently, unless you are sure of the diagnosis, and that active intervention is inappropriate.

Initial management

- Assessment and diagnosis must proceed at the same time as resuscitation.
- Secure the airway (recovery position, airway adjuncts, e.g. oropharyngeal).
- Intubate if need be:
  - Respiration may deteriorate suddenly
  - Intubation protects the airway against aspirating vomit
  - Perform a rapid neurological examination first if sedation is required.
- Initially give oxygen by trauma mask.
- Monitor pulse, BP, and respiratory rate and pattern, pulse oximetry, and/or arterial blood gases. Adjust oxygen to keep oxygen saturation >95%.
- Check blood glucose. If low (<3mmol/L), give 50mL 20% glucose IV (plus B vitamins/Pabrinex® IV if alcoholic or malnourished).
- Terminate seizures with IV lorazepam (2mg repeated twice if necessary) or IV diazepam (10mg, repeated twice if necessary). If no IV access use rectal diazepam. If seizures persist, or for maintenance, use IV phenytoin (loading dose 15mg/kg at <50mg/min with ECG monitoring, then 100mg tds).
- Rapid neurological examination:
  - Hand drop over head (to exclude malingering)
  - Neck stiffness (unless cervical spine trauma possible)
  - Pupil size and reactivity to light
  - Eye movement assessment (doll's eyes manoeuvre)
  - Response to painful stimulus (knuckle to sternum, nail bed pressure)
  - Limb tone, movement, and plantar responses.
- Take blood for blood count, biochemistry, including calcium, renal, thyroid, and liver function, and lactate.
- Start IV normal saline (1L over 8h, unless clinically hypovolaemic, or in overt heart failure).
- Insert a urinary catheter only if you need urine for toxicology screening, or to measure urine output.
- Treat hyperthermia (tepid sponge) or hypothermia (space blanket, Bair Hugger®).
- If overdose is suspected, consult toxbase (🕮 www.toxbase.org) for instructions.
- Arrange urgent CT head.
- Monitor conscious level using the GCS.

Presumed supratentorial mass lesions with raised intracranial pressure

- Intubate and hyperventilate to lower intracranial pressure in the short term (30min to a few hours, by vasoconstricting and reducing intracerebral blood volume).
- Tilt head up (30 degrees).
- Give 20% mannitol 0.5–1g/kg (about 250mL), over 15min (reduces intracranial pressure in 20–60min and lasts 4–6h). Usually a short-term measure whilst a diagnosis is made. Monitor blood electrolytes.
- If stroke is the cause, hyperventilation and mannitol are not particularly effective.
- Give dexamethasone 4mg IV (6-hourly) if CT head shows vasogenic oedema secondary to tumour or abscess. Effective in several hours. Ineffective in stroke.
- Refer to a neurosurgeon if a tumour, abscess, or hydrocephalus is diagnosed, and consider referral if there is a haematoma or malignant middle cerebral artery infarction (see 📖 Hemicraniectomy, p.44).

Infratentorial lesions

- Reduce intracranial pressure as described earlier.
- Refer to neurosurgeon for decompression of cerebellar haematoma, or cerebellar infarct with oedema.
- Treat intrinsic brain stem tumours with dexamethasone in the first instance.

Toxic or metabolic coma

- Exclude or treat hypoglycaemia.
- Severe metabolic acidosis (pH <7.0) give IV sodium bicarbonate 1mmol/kg (1.26% is 150mmol/L and can be given peripherally).
- If carbon monoxide poisoning give 100% oxygen (consider transfer to hyperbaric oxygen facility).
- If CT normal, consider a lumbar puncture.
- If history, signs, or CSF suggest acute bacterial meningitis, treat according to local microbiological advice.
- Drug overdose—mainly supportive, but specific antidotes may help:
  - Contact a specialist toxicology centre for advice (e.g. 🕸 http://www.toxbase.org)
  - Opiates—naloxone IV 400mcg repeated at 2-min intervals up to maximum 10mg. Short duration of action, and may need repeating or infusing.
  - Benzodiazepines—flumazenil 200mcg IV, then 100mcg at 60-s intervals, if required, maximum dose 1mg. Short-acting and may need repeating or infusing (100–400mcg/h). Response can be dramatic, but avoid if also taken tricyclic antidepressants (risk of seizures).

Acute medical management of cerebral infarcts

Strategies include:

- Diagnostic accuracy and aetiological understanding.
- Reperfusion (thrombolysis).
- Physiological normalization (controlling BP, maintaining oxygenation, normalizing blood glucose, reducing pyrexia, fluid rehydration).
- Prevention, or early detection and treatment, of neurological and medical complications.

Diagnosis should be reviewed by a senior clinician with expertise in stroke within 24h of admission, and sooner if necessary.

Most recommendations are likely to be of benefit on a balance of probabilities rather than proven beyond doubt in randomized trials.

Thrombolysis

Thrombolysis can reduce death and disability, but only if given to highly selected patients who can reach hospital, be assessed, have a CT scan, and treatment started within 4.5h (Boxes 2.3 and 2.4). One patient is saved from death or dependency for every 10 thrombolysed. For centres giving thrombolysis, target 'door-to-needle time' is <1h.

- Thrombolysis with IV recombinant tissue plasminogen activator (tPA, alteplase; 0.9mg/kg, maximum 90mg, 10% as bolus, rest over 1h) in the absence of contraindications.
- 📖 Appendices 5–7, pp.328–332, give details of medical work-up, a suitability checklist, and monitoring requirements.

The risk is doing more harm than good. Symptomatic intracranial haemorrhages occur in 6% after thrombolysis compared with 1% with placebo. The hospital must have the staffing and infrastructure to deliver thrombolysis safely to an agreed protocol. There is a long list of contra-indications and cautions, and monitoring must be rigorous.

Be cautious, but not overcautious. Severe strokes, including those with extensive early changes on CT scan (e.g. more than a third of the MCA territory involved), do badly regardless of treatment, but may do less badly if treated. Similarly 'minor' neurological deficits (e.g. aphasia, hemianopia) can have a major impact if they do not recover, justifying treatment. 'Protocol violation' is associated with increased haemorrhage rates, but a critical review of contraindications suggested that not all of these are well-justified.[1]

Intra-arterial thrombolysis, or mechanical clot retrieval, for proximal MCA occlusion within 6h of onset, is similarly effective where interventional neuroradiological expertise is available.

Basilar artery thrombosis has a poor prognosis if untreated. If symptoms are progressing, and a basilar artery thrombosis has been demonstrated radiologically, consider intra-arterial thrombolysis if there is sufficient local expertise (interventional neuroradiologists). Some case series suggest that mortality is halved (to about 40%) by thrombolysis. Intervention can be up to 12h or more from stroke onset. Use IV thrombolysis if the patient otherwise fulfils treatment criteria. Otherwise anticoagulate with heparin. By the time progression has reached coma and quadriparesis, survival is unlikely.

Reference

1 De Keyser J et al. Intravenous alteplase for stroke: beyond the guidelines and in particular clinical situations. Stroke 2007; **38**:2612–18.

Box 2.3 Trials of tPA (alteplase) in acute stroke

- The National Institute of Neurological Disorders and Stroke (NINDS) trial randomized 624 patients to 0.9mg/kg tPA or placebo, half within 90min of stroke and half within 180min. After 3 months there was a small benefit with thrombolysis on a 42-point neurological score, the NIH Stroke Scale (median scores 8 vs 12), and a small reduction in mortality (17% vs 21%, p=0.30). More patients had complete or almost complete recovery on four outcome scales, including the Rankin scale (43% vs 27%). 13–16% had a more favourable 3-month outcome with tPA compared with placebo.
- The European Co-operative Acute Stroke Study (ECASS) randomized 620 patients to 1.1mg/kg tPA or placebo, within 6h of stroke onset. There was a small benefit for tPA in neurological and functional outcomes, at the cost of an increased mortality rate. 30-day mortality was 18% vs 13%, but 36% of the tPA group were independent on the Rankin Scale vs 29% for placebo (scores 0–1; OR 1.2, 95% CI 0.98–1.35).
- ECASS-2 randomized 800 patients to 0.9mg/kg tPA or placebo within 6h of stroke onset. Strokes were less severe than those in ECASS. 11% of patients died within 90 days in each group. There was a small advantage for tPA over placebo (40% vs 37% for Rankin scores 0–1, or 54% vs 46% for Rankin scores 0–2).
- Data from 2775 patients randomized in these trials (plus the ATLANTIS trials) have been pooled and re-analysed. The outcome was full, or nearly full, recovery defined by the Rankin (0–1), NIHSS (0–1) or Barthel (>95/100) scores after 3 months. Benefit from treatment decreased with time from stroke onset. For treatment within 0–90min, OR for favourable outcomes was 2.8 (95% CI 1.8–4.5), for 91–180min 1.6 (1.1–2.2), for 181–270min 1.4 (0.1–1.9), and for 271–360min 1.2 (0.9–1.5).
- Another overview estimated a relative risk for death or dependency of 0.66 (95% CI 0.53–0.83) for patients treated within 3h, absolute risk reduction 50% vs 60% (95% CI for difference 5–16%, number needed to treat [NNT] 10). 6% of thrombolysed patients experienced intracerebral bleeds, half fatal, compared to 1% for placebo.
- ECASS-3 randomized 800 patients to 0.9mg/kg tPA or placebo between 3 and 4.5 h after stroke onset (median 3h 59min). Strokes were less severe than in ECASS-2. 7.7% vs 8.4% of patients died within 90 days. There was a small advantage for tPA over placebo (52% vs 45% for Rankin scores 0–1, or 67% vs 62% for Rankin scores 0–2), in line with that expected from the pooled analysis (OR 1.3, 95% CI 1.0–1.8). Symptomatic intracranial haemorrhage rate was 2.4% vs 0.2% (about the same as in other trials, but using a different definition).

Lancet 2004; **363**:768–74.
New England Journal of Medicine 2008; **359**:1317–29.

Box 2.4 Health-care system requirements for delivering thrombolysis

- *Public knowledge*: acute onset of focal neurological signs prompts emergency attendance at hospital or calling an ambulance ('FAST' test, see 📖 Box 2.2, p.35).
- *General practitioners*: direct acute focal neurology to hospital immediately.
- *Ambulance service*: priority attendance at calls and transfer to hospital, oxygenation and IV hydration, blood sugar check, question witnesses for time of onset, direct admission to acute stroke unit, advance warning of arrival at hospital.
- *Hospital emergency department*: initiate assessment, alert acute stroke team, order emergency CT scan, IV access, blood tests sent.
- *CT scanner and reporting*: 24-h immediate access. Follow up CT scan availability for complications. Immediate reliable reporting of scans by radiologist or stroke physician/neurologist.
- *On-call stroke or neurological team*:
  - Work-up (📖 Appendix 5, p.328), blood tests reviewed
  - Medical stabilization
  - Head scan interpretation
  - Complete suitability checklist (📖 Appendix 6, p.330)
  - Consent (or assessment of best interests)
  - Immediate access to tPA.
- *Ward*: monitoring facilities and trained staff (📖 Appendix 7, p.332).
- *Governance*: monitoring and audit of indications, process, complications, and outcomes.

Other acute medical management

Guidelines for immediate medical treatment and management of specific neurological complications are given in Table 2.2.

Table 2.2 Acute treatment for physiological normalization

Abnormality	Intervention
Fluid balance	IV saline infusion, central venous pressure 8–10cm H_2O. Less if raised intracranial pressure
Low BP (<140/90mmHg)	Control arrhythmias. Stop antihypertensive drugs. IV fluids to maintain filling pressure, target BP 160–180/90–100mmHg
Sustained high BP >220/120mmHg, after 1st hour	Reduce slowly to 180/105mmHg with oral ACEI, IV labetolol in 10-mg doses up to 150mg, or IV nitrates (isosorbide dinitrate 1–10mg/h). Avoid sublingual nifedipine
Mild–moderate hypoxia	2–4L/min O_2 by mask or nasal cannulae, keep SaO_2 >95%
Severe hypoxia, unconscious	Intubation and ventilation if need be (taking account of prognosis, comorbidity and patient's wishes)
Glucose >10mmol/L	IV insulin sliding scale, reduce to 4–10mmol/L (see Box 2.5)
Pyrexia >37.5°C	Investigate source. Antibiotics if evidence of infection; paracetamol 1g PO/PR/IV qds
Comorbid conditions	Optimize
Raised intracranial pressure	Mild dehydration, head up 30 degrees, 20% mannitol, consider decompressive craniotomy for extensive MCA or cerebellar infarction

Box 2.5 Euglycaemia after stroke—GIST trial[1]

- 899 patients within 24h of acute stroke, and with glucose 6–17mmol/L were randomized between euglycaemia (4–7mmol/L) using a glucose–potassium–insulin (GKI) infusion for 24h, or control (saline infusion). Intended sample size was 2355; the trial terminated early due to slow recruitment.
- Median glucose at entry was 7.6 (IQR 6.7–9.0) mmol/L. On treatment glucose fell to 6.1–6.6mmol/L in the GKI group and 6.8mmol/L in the control group, a mean difference of 0.6mmol/L. Mean BP was 9mmHg lower in the GKI group (an effect of potassium and insulin).
- Relative risks with active GKI treatment were:
  - 1.14 (95% CI 0.86–1.51) for death (30% vs 27%)
  - 1.02 (95% CI 0.90–1.15) for death or severe dependency (Rankin scale >3; 54% vs 53%).
- An impairment score, the European Stroke Severity Score was the same at 90 days (73 vs 75, p=0.6).
- There were no differences for patients treated within 6h, nor for those treated per protocol.
- Unfortunately this trial tested too small an intervention (reduction of glucose by 0.6mmol/L), in too few participants (899/2355 intended), who were at barely increased risk due to hyperglycaemia (median glucose at entry 7.6mmol/L). The question of whether reducing raised glucose improves outcomes remains completely open, and in the absence of likely harm, restoring euglycaemia remains reasonable management.

Lancet Neurology 2007; **6**:397–406.

Blood pressure

Cerebral autoregulation is lost in areas of evolving infarction, so blood flow is passively dependent on mean arterial pressure. The first objective after stroke is to avoid drops in BP. An arbitrary upper limit of 220/120mmHg is set by some, with the proviso that BP reduction should be slow, <25%, and not go below target (180/100mmHg) in the first 24h. The objectives of BP lowering are to avoid cerebral oedema and reduce the chances of vessel rupture (which is proportional to mean arterial pressure, so small reductions only marginally reduce risk).

Observational evidence suggests best outcomes are with initial systolic pressures of 140–180mmHg, which corresponds to recommendations made based on cerebral blood flow.

Existing antihypertensive medication can be continued, but should be stopped if BP is below target. BP should not be reduced in the first hour, unless there is:

- High BP post thrombolysis (see 📖 Appendix 5, p.328).
- Hypertensive encephalopathy (very high BP, headache, visual disturbance, drowsiness and confusion, seizures, retinopathy, and papilloedema).
- Hypertensive heart failure or acute MI.
- Acute renal failure.

- Aortic dissection.
- Eclampsia or pre-eclampsia.

Aspirin

Aspirin, given early when bleeding is excluded or unlikely, has proven long-term benefit, but the effect is small (Box 2.6). 80 patients must be treated to prevent one patient suffering death or dependency. If you don't treat the patient in front of you, he or she is unlikely to come to much harm. However, applied across the UK to, say, 60 000 suitable ischaemic stroke patients per year, 750 will be saved from death or dependency.

- Give aspirin 150–300mg orally or rectally, thereafter 75mg per day orally (or 300mg rectally), except where chances of haemorrhage are clinically thought to be high (loss of consciousness, headache, vomiting). In the UK, NICE recommends 300mg for the first 2 weeks, but the evidence supporting this is weak.

Box 2.6 International Stroke Trial (IST) and Chinese Acute Stroke Trial (CAST)

- *IST*: 20 000 patients with acute stroke (within 48h) randomized to aspirin (300mg/day or placebo), and heparin (25 000IU/day or 10 000IU/day or placebo), in a 2×3 factorial design, for 14 days, or discharge if sooner.
- *CAST*: 21 100 patients randomized to 160mg/day of aspirin or placebo for 4 weeks or until discharged.
- *Aspirin*: small reduction in risk of death, dependency, or recurrent stroke. In IST, deaths within 14 days were 9.0% vs 9.4% (risk ratio 0.96); death or recurrent strokes were 11.3% vs 12.4% (risk ratio 0.91); death or dependency at 6 months were 62.2% vs 63.5% (risk ratio 0.98, NNT 77). No subgroup benefited significantly more or less. In CAST, deaths were 3.9% vs to 3.3% (risk ratio 0.85); death or non-fatal stroke 5.9% vs 5.3% (risk ratio 0.89); death or dependency 31.6% vs 30.5% (risk ratio 0.97). Pooled odds ratios for death or non-fatal stroke were 0.89 (95% CI 0.83–0.95), and for death or dependency were 0.95 (95% CI 0.91–0.99) in favour of aspirin treatment. There was a small excess of cerebral bleeds on aspirin (1.01% vs 0.83%).
- *Heparin*: no difference in the number of deaths within 14 days—9.0% vs 9.3% (risk ratio 0.97); and death or dependency at 6 months was 62.9% in each group. Fewer recurrent ischaemic strokes were balanced by an increase in haemorrhagic strokes. The lower dose of heparin was associated with fewer deaths and non-fatal strokes than the higher dose, but there was no advantage in the death or dependence end-point at 6 months. No subgroup, including 3000 patients with AF, benefited significantly more than the average.

Lancet 1997; **349**:1569–81.
Lancet 1997; **349**:1641–9.

Anticoagulation

Anticoagulation is unlikely to be beneficial in most acute strokes, including those associated with AF (Box 2.6). In some situations anticoagulation is sensible, including:

- An underanticoagulated patient with a mechanical heart valve.
- Vertebral or carotid arterial dissection.
- Basilar artery thrombosis.
- Venous sinus thrombosis.

Anticoagulation with heparin (5000IU IV, then 15–25IU/kg/h, and check APTT after 4–6h then daily, or 4–6h after a dose change) is more reversible than low-molecular-weight heparins (LMWHs), so might be safer if there is bleeding. LMWHs are less prone to under- or overcoagulation. There is no hard evidence to guide the choice.

In arterial dissection, aspirin is a reasonable alternative if there is good reason to avoid anticoagulation (e.g. extracranial bleeding, intracranial dissection).

In suspected basilar artery thrombosis, anticoagulate with heparin pending imaging (MR or conventional angiography) and consideration of intra-arterial thrombolysis.

Prophylactic-dose LMWH (or low-dose heparin 5000IU bd subcutaneously), prevents deep vein thromboses (DVTs), but does not alter outcomes overall (see 🕮 Box 2.6, p.43). Consider it for patients at high risk (e.g. severely immobile, history of venous thromboembolism, or severe overweight). Otherwise use hydration, aspirin, and early mobilization to reduce risk. Antiembolism compression stockings are ineffective (see 🕮 Box 2.9, p.54).

Hemicraniectomy

Large MCA infarcts in younger adults can result in so called 'malignant infarction'. Swelling of the infarct, usually maximal between the 2nd and 5th days after onset, in the absence of age-related cerebral atrophy, can result in mass effect, with greatly raised intracranial pressure, midline shift, and coning (Fig. 2.1).

Hemicraniectomy is the raising of a large bone flap from the skull vault, to allow release of pressure. People with large infarcts tend to do badly, both for survival and recovery of function. The worry was that this technique might lead to more severely-disabled survivors. However, trials demonstrate that mortality is reduced, and chances of good recovery are increased, by hemicraniectomy, although the risk of surviving with severe disability remains (Box 2.7).

Consult a neurosurgeon if:
- The patient is <60 years old
- MCA infarction is confirmed on CT scan

- Level of consciousness is impaired and decreasing
- Within 24–48h of onset.

If this procedure is being contemplated, interventions to lower intracranial pressure in the short term (such as mannitol, or intubation and hyperventilation) are sensible, while arrangements for surgery are made.

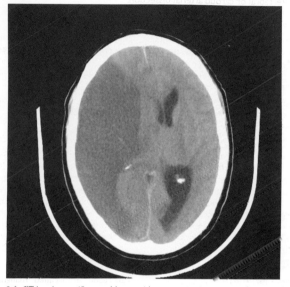

Fig. 2.1 CT head scan. 45 year old man with progressive drowsiness after a stroke. 'Malignant' MCA territory infarction.

Box 2.7 Hemicraniectomy for malignant MCA territory infarction

- Up to 10% of cerebral infarcts are associated with severe mass effect due to swelling, with midline shift, depressed conscious level, and up to 80% mortality. Case series of hemicraniectomy with duraplasty suggested dramatic reduction in mortality, with a reasonable prospect of functional recovery.
- Data from three small randomized trials (Destiny, Decimal, and Hamlet) were pooled.
- 93 participants, aged 18–60 years, with NIHSS score >15, depressed level of consciousness, CT evidence of >50% MCA territory infarction, or MRI DWI lesion >145mL were randomized between hemicraniectomy and best medical management, within 48h of ischaemic stroke (mean 24h).
- Outcomes were based on the modified Rankin Scale (mRS) after 1 year: 0–1, no disability; 2, slight disability, being unable to carry out all previous activities, but able to look after own affairs without assistance; 3, moderate disability, requiring some help, but being able to walk without assistance; 4, moderately severe disability, being unable to walk without assistance and unable to attend to own bodily needs without assistance; 5, severe disability, being bedridden, incontinent, and requiring constant nursing care and attention; 6, death. Given stroke severity, in this context, mRS=3 represents a good outcome.
- Relative risks for operated patients were:
  - 0.10 (95% CI 0.04–0.27) for mortality at 6 months (22% vs 71%)
  - 0.10 (95% CI 0.04–0.27) for combined death or severe disability (mRS 5–6; 26% vs 76%)
  - 3.0 (95% CI 1.2–7.7) for survival with mild–moderate disability (mRS 0–3; 43% vs 21%)
  - 4.9 (95% CI 1.6–15.6) for moderate to severe disability (mRS 4–5; 35% vs 7%).
- Chances of survival and good recovery are increased by hemicraniectomy, but at the cost of a greater chance of survival with moderate to severe disability. Without operation, of every 10 patients 7 die, 1 is moderately to severely disabled, and 2 make a reasonable recovery. With operation, 2 die, 4 are moderately to severely disabled, and 4 make a reasonable recovery.
- Extrapolation of findings outside of the restrictive inclusion criteria for this analysis remains uncertain (e.g. age over 60, time after 48h).

Lancet Neurology 2007; **6**:215–22.

Acute management of intracerebral haemorrhage

- Haematomas expand over the first few hours after onset. Preventing this expansion (e.g. by reversing anticoagulation) may reduce primary brain damage.
- Logically, evacuation of the haematoma should help, but the one large trial of this found no benefit. However, it did not exclude the possibility of benefit in some subgroups (Box 2.8). Conservative management is reasonable, but neurosurgeons may attempt evacuation, especially in a younger patient, with a superficial bleed and no more than moderate depression of consciousness, when an underlying aneurysm is suspected, or when an initially-well patient is deteriorating. Consult early.
- Cerebellar haematoma is an exception, where evacuation may be life-saving and the prospects for good functional recovery are reasonable. Surgery is particularly indicated if level of consciousness is impaired, and haematoma volume is >40mL (3cm diameter), or if there is hydrocephalus or brain stem compression.
- Prognosis is poor when consciousness is lost, and hopeless if there is no response to pain and absent brainstem reflexes for a few hours.
- The mainstay of treatment, as with cerebral infarcts, is to optimize brain perfusion and oxygenation by supporting cardiorespiratory function (oxygen, fluids to maintain BP), limiting other damaging physiological abnormalities (pyrexia, hyperglycaemia), and preventing or aggressively treating systemic complications.
- There is little evidence to support reducing high BP. For the time being we suggest reduction only at very high levels (>230/120mmHg), and to modest extent (mean 25% or no lower than 180/100mmHg in the first 24h). Some guidelines support modest BP lowering (e.g. American Heart Association guidelines suggest reducing systolic BP if >180 mmHg, to a target of 160/90mmHg, or cerebral perfusion pressure of 60–80mmHg if intracranial pressure is monitored). UK NICE guidelines make no recommendation on reducing BP. A 400-patient pilot trial of BP reduction after acute haemorrhage suggested that treatment was safe, but did not demonstrate improved outcomes. Any BP reduction would have to start very soon (within 3–6h, ideally within 1h) after onset to be effective in preventing haematoma expansion. The greater danger may be from low BP compromising cerebral perfusion.
- Prothrombotic drugs (e.g. recombinant factor VII) are of no benefit.

Box 2.8 Surgical intervention for acute intracerebral haemorrhage—STICH trial

- 1083 patients with acute primary supratentorial intracerebral haemorrhage within 72h of onset were randomized to surgery to evacuate the haematoma (mean time of surgery 30h after onset), or medical management (although 26% of this group went on to have surgical evacuation, at a mean of 60h after onset).
- Patients were randomized if their surgeon felt uncertain about whether evacuation would be beneficial or not.
- The outcome was disability at 6 months (adjusted for initial prognosis, so that those with the worst prognosis were deemed to have had a good outcome with a greater degree of disability than those with an initial better prognosis).
- Relative risk for surgery was:
  - 0·89 (95% CI 0·66–1·19) for good outcomes (26% vs 24%)
  - 0.95 (95% CI 0.73-1.23) for mortality (36% vs 37%).
- No subgroup was clearly different from the whole trial population. Patients with superficial haematomas, and those with an initial GCS score of 9–12 had outcomes better than the average, but no more so than could have occurred by chance. Those presenting in coma (GCS <9) fared almost uniformly badly.
- This trial gives no support for surgical intervention after acute intracerebral haemorrhage. Undertaking this trial was a Herculean effort, logistically and culturally. But it is important to realize that it cannot exclude the possibility that surgery is beneficial for some patients. Maybe surgeons can spot those who will benefit from surgery. In which case those who stood to benefit most from surgery were not randomized. The trial was underpowered to detect differences reliably between surgery and medical management in important subgroups. And if surgery were beneficial, the trial results would have been diluted by the rate of delayed surgery in the medically managed group.

Lancet 2005; **365**:387–97.

Anticoagulated patients with intracerebral haemorrhage

- The risk of bleeding to life and health outweighs the risk from clotting in the short term.
- Consult a haematologist urgently:
  - If on warfarin, reverse the anticoagulation *immediately* (within the hour) with prothrombin complex concentrate (PCC) (factors II, VII, IX, and X; Beriplex® 50U/kg IV) plus 10mg vitamin K IV. PCC achieves reversal of anticoagulation better and quicker than fresh frozen plasma, but if this is all that is available give 15mL/kg IV.
  - If on heparin, stop infusion. Reverse with protamine sulphate (1mg/100U heparin received in last 3h; initial 10-mg test dose IV over 10min, observe for anaphylaxis; if stable give entire calculated dose slowly over 10min; maximum dose 50mg). A lower dose is needed as time from heparin administration increases, e.g. half dose only 30min after infusion stopped.
  - If on LMWH (e.g. enoxaparin, dalteparin), only 60% of anti-Xa activity is reversed by protamine. There is no other antidote.
  - If thrombolysed, give fibrinogen concentrate (or cryoprecipitate), and platelets (if <100 × 10^9/L). Check fibrinogen level, if <1g/L give more. Antifibrinolytics (aprotinin or tranexamic acid) probably don't help.
  - Factor VIII if haemophiliac.
  - Platelets if thrombocytopenic (<80 × 10^9/L; in immune thrombocytopenia immune suppression is also required, but this will take at least 24h to be effective).
- If the patient has a mechanical heart valve, it is safe to discontinue anticoagulation for 2–4 weeks, both for aortic and mitral valves (the daily risk of valve failure or embolism off anticoagulation is <0.02%).

How long for?

Continue physiological normalization until the patient is stable. With minor strokes, aggressive IV therapy may not be required at all. Patients with moderate or severe strokes are unstable (i.e. liable to deteriorate) over a week or more. Judge each patient's needs day-to-day depending on the circumstances, such as level of consciousness and ability to swallow. Generally we suggest continuing supportive measures for 2–7 days.

Acute nursing care

Recognize two complementary roles, one or other of which may predominate, but which often go on together:
- Supportive, active, 'doing for' care, in severe acute illness.
- Encouraging, enabling, progressive withdrawal of support to promote independence.

This section concentrates on the acute supportive role.

Maintain airway

Nurse in the coma position if unconscious. An airway adjunct or intubation may be necessary.

Maintain oxygenation

- The ultimate size of the infarct may depend on maintaining adequate oxygen delivery to ischaemic brain.
- Keep oxygen saturation >95%. Give oxygen if necessary, unless contraindicated, by mask or nasal cannulae. Monitor by pulse oximetry.
- Stop oxygen and call for medical reassessment if respiratory rate drops below 10/min, or if desaturation (<92%) occurs on oxygen (indicating that respiratory drive may be dependent on hypoxia, sometimes seen in chronic obstructive pulmonary disease).

Avoid pressure sores

- These can arise in as little as 30min when a severely immobile patient is placed on a sufficiently hard surface. They can develop in Emergency and Radiology departments, as well as on wards. Vulnerable sites are the sacrum, greater trochanters (hips), and heels. Sores are painful, debilitating, and unpleasant. A deep sore takes many months to heal, consuming expensive materials, and scarce nursing time.
- Complete a pressure sore risk score immediately on admission, and certainly within 4h (e.g. Waterlow). Most sores are avoidable with sufficient attention to pressure relief. Avoidance by turning alone is labour intensive.
- Pressure relieving mattresses (and cushions for chairs) should be immediately available 24h a day. These cannot prevent all sores, and a turning regimen is also required. Additional attention is needed to prevent heel sores.
- Reassess risk every 24h.

Hydration and nutrition

- Swallowing is not safe initially in about half of stroke patients admitted to hospital. Nurses (and doctors) should be able to make a simple assessment of whether swallowing is safe or not. The patient must be sitting up, and conscious level sufficient to allow cooperation:
  - Give a sip (5–10mL) of water, using a teaspoon if necessary.
  - Observe for failure to seal the lips.
  - Look/feel for prompt laryngeal elevation indicating swallowing.
  - Record if it is delayed or incomplete.

- Observe for choking, coughing, or a 'wet' quality to the voice, indicating fluid around the vocal cords.
  - If all appears well, repeat twice, and then try a larger volume.
  - Then observe whilst eating their first meal for coughing or choking, chewing problems, loss of food from lips, or inability to move food in the mouth (pouching).
  - At the same time check for mouth dryness or other mouth care needs.
- You cannot swallow with your neck extended. Positioning is therefore very important—sitting up, or leaning slightly forward.
- If swallowing is not safe:
  - Do not give anything by mouth.
  - Make plans for mouth care.
  - Hydrate intravenously, and consider nasogastric feeding.
  - Repeat the swallow assessment at least daily.
  - Refer to a speech and language therapist if still unsafe on day 2–3, and the patient is alert and well enough to cooperate.
- IV hydration may also be required to maintain an optimal BP (systolic pressure >140mmHg).
- Nasogastric tubes:
  - Use one if oral intake is inadequate by day 2, so long as death is not thought to be imminent, and your best information is that the patient would have wanted you to do so.
  - You may need one earlier, e.g. to administer medication.
  - Many people find these uncomfortable or irritating, and they are often dislodged or pulled out. A loop or 'bridle' secured behind the nasal septum can help.
  - They disrupt oesophageal peristalsis and cardiac sphincter function, are associated with gastro-oesophageal reflux and increase the risk of aspiration.
  - However, they can deliver adequate nutrition in many cases.

Antivenous thrombosis prophylaxis

- Aspirin, good hydration, and early mobilization all help prevent DVTs.
- Prophylactic dose LMWH (e.g. enoxaparin) prevents DVTs, but does not alter outcomes overall. Consider it if patient is at high risk (e.g. severely immobile, history of venous thromboembolism, severe overweight).
- Graduated compression stockings are ineffective at preventing DVTs, and can cause skin problems (Box 2.9).

Box 2.9 Graduated thigh length compression stocking fail to prevent DVT in immobile patients after stroke

- 2518 patients admitted to hospital within 1 week of an acute stroke, and who were immobile, were randomized to routine care plus thigh-length graduated compression stockings (n=1256), or to routine care plus avoidance of stockings (n=1262).
- Compression Doppler ultrasound of both legs was done at 7–10 days and 25–30 days. Primary outcome was symptomatic or asymptomatic DVT in the popliteal or femoral veins.
- Relative risk when wearing stockings was:
  - 0.95 (95% CI 0.76–1.20) for DVT (10.0% vs 10.5%)
  - 4·2 (95% CI 2·4–7·3) for skin breaks, ulcers, blisters, and skin necrosis (5% vs 1%).
- Data do not support the use of thigh-length graduated compression stockings in patients admitted to hospital with acute stroke. But the study could not exclude up to a 24% relative risk reduction whilst wearing stockings.

*Lancet 2009; **373**:1958–65.*

Positioning and support

A positioning and handling plan is required as part of the initial nursing and physiotherapy assessments.
- The aim of early intervention is:
  - To prevent abnormal tone, contractures, and pressure sores.
  - To maintain correct alignment of body parts to make normal movement patterns possible or easier.
  - To avoid the establishment of abnormal patterns.
- Distinguish between:
  - Comfort positioning (for agitated or dying patients).
  - Therapeutic positioning (which maximizes the chances of future recovery and function).
- Prolonged supine lying (on the back) increases extensor spasticity and should be avoided unless comfort is the priority:
  - Place a pillow under the head and affected shoulder.
  - Legs should lie symmetrically.
- Side lying is preferred (Figs. 2.2 and 2.3):
  - Support the head on one pillow.
  - The trunk should be straight.
  - Bring the hemiplegic arm out in front of the patient, extended if underneath, slightly flexed if on top.
  - Make sure the shoulder is forward so that the weight is slightly behind the shoulder tip.
  - Extend the hemiplegic leg, and flex the unaffected leg to give support. Don't support under the foot (to dorsiflex it), as this can stimulate extensor activity.
  - Support the upper arm, leg and back with pillows.

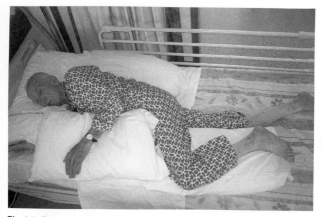

Fig. 2.2 Correct positioning, left hemiparesis, lying on the unaffected side.

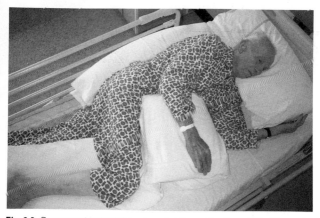

Fig. 2.3 Correct positioning, left hemiparesis, lying on the affected side. The trunk is straight. The shoulder is forward and the hemiplegic arm in front of the patient. The hemiplegic leg is extended. The head, trunk and upper arm are supported by pillows.

- If sitting in bed (Fig. 2.4):
  - Keep upright and symmetrical.
  - Supported on both sides.
  - A pillow under the hemiplegic forearm.

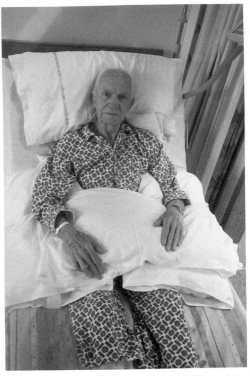

Fig. 2.4 Correct positioning, sitting in bed (e.g. for feeding). The trunk is upright and symmetrical, supported on both sides, a pillow under the affected arm. There is additional support behind the affected shoulder.

- When sitting in a chair (Fig. 2.5):
  - The hip, knees, and ankle should be at right angles.
  - Feet flat on the floor.
  - Keep the hip well-aligned, as it will tend to fall into external rotation.
  - Sitting should be symmetrical (equal weight on each buttock).
  - Support the trunk on both sides with pillows or rolled towels, or use specialist trunk supports or chairs (e.g. Wolfston, Hydrotilt) to keep the patient relaxed.
  - The paralysed arm should be supported on a pillow, placed forward (shoulder slightly flexed), close to the trunk, and in neutral rotation or slightly externally rotated, with the elbow in neutral flexion/extension.

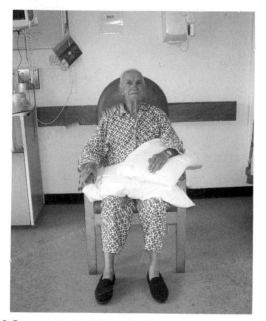

Fig. 2.5 Correct positioning, sitting in a chair. Sitting is symmetrical, bottom well back in the chair. Feet are flat on the floor. The hip, knee, and ankle are at right angles, and well aligned. Affected arm is supported on a pillow.

The affected shoulder

Take care with it. Damage may be done very early on. Shoulder pain can be very persistent (see 📖 Shoulder pain, p.200 and Box 8.5, p.201).
- There is often insufficient muscle activity to support the joint in its correct position. Incorrect handling can sublux the joint and damage the joint capsule.
- When the patient is sitting:
  - Support the arm with a pillow to keep the humerus in a neutral position and close to the body.
  - Keep the wrist and fingers straight.
  - Don't ignore an arm hanging over the side of the bed or chair.
- Support the arm under the shoulder when moving it away from the body, and limit movement away from the body to 30° at most.
- Patients and relatives should be taught the importance of shoulder care, and to challenge health or social care staff if they are about to perform a potentially damaging manoeuvre.
- Encourage the patient to hold or support his or her own arm at the wrist when transferring or standing.
- When lying on the affected side, ease the shoulder forward so the patient's weight is slightly behind the shoulder tip.
- Never pull on the affected arm.
- Encourage active movement.
- Discourage gripping activities (they promote abnormal tone).

Transferring

The primary aim is to avoid injuries to the patient (shoulder, falls) and staff (back and neck), which have been unfortunately common in the past. Transferring is also a therapeutic opportunity:
- Like all practical physical skills, you cannot learn this from a book. You need proper training and supervised practice.
- A manual handling assessment should be made as soon as possible after admission, and certainly within 12h.
  - Take account of alertness, communication, cognition, vision, and previous ability.
  - You must have access to appropriate transferring aids.
  - If there is doubt about safety, a physiotherapist should assess and advise.
- The transfer will not work unless the patient can stand safely, and can engage in active cooperation.
- Beware a patient who tries to grab you as he or she stands.
- A patient who pushes to one side during a transfer is likely to slip or overbalance.
- Use an aid if the transfer is difficult. If in doubt, always choose the safer option.
- If necessary, use a hoist. It will do the job, but is slow and non-therapeutic.
- A standing hoist encourages some standing.
- A rotunda involves standing, but encourages overuse of the unaffected side, and poor-quality standing alignment.

- 'Banana' (sliding) boards can be used for (sitting) bed–chair transfers, and encourage participation.
- Transfer with a Zimmer or rollator frame only after a physiotherapy assessment.

Bladder and bowel management

- 60% of patients admitted with stroke will be initially incontinent of urine.
- An early assessment of the likely cause of incontinence should always be made including:
  - Dipstick urinalysis.
  - Post-void residual volume (by ultrasound scan).
  - Ascertaining previous bladder and bowel problems.
- Indwelling urethral catheters always cause problems, including infection, blockage, bladder spasm, and urethral trauma. They are best avoided:
  - If there is retention, intermittent catheterization is preferable.
  - A sheath catheter or incontinence pads should be able to keep the skin dry, and contain wetness adequately.
  - However, for patients with drowsiness, severe immobility, absent sitting balance, or developing skin problems, it is hard to argue that a catheter is never an acceptable means of containment in the short term, so long as the decision is constantly reviewed.

Explanation and reassurance

The patient is likely to be frightened and bewildered, especially if aphasic. Relatives may be as well.

Monitoring

Monitoring should be:
- Individually tailored to meet the circumstances of the individual patient.
- Reviewed regularly, so scarce nursing and medical time is not wasted with unnecessary observations.
- Prioritized—it may be necessary to compromise on the ideal, if other important tasks (rehabilitation nursing, counselling) are neglected because of time spent on 'monitoring'.

A thrombolysed patient requires high-dependency monitoring (Ⅲ Appendix 7, p.332). Otherwise, the following parameters should be considered acutely:
- Neurological status:
  - Level of consciousness—the GCS (see Ⅲ Appendix 3, p.325) is well-established and familiar, and changes of >3 points, or a gradually declining score require explanation and/or action.
  - Progression of neurological impairments. This can be by serial traditional neurological examination, or using a stroke severity scale, such as the Scandinavian or National Institutes of Health (NIH) stroke scales (Ⅲ Appendices 8 and 9, pp 334, 338)
- Cardiovascular status: pulse and BP, 4-hourly initially. May be required more often if unstable.
- Respiratory: pulse oximetry.
- Temperature.
- Blood glucose (by glucometer), if diabetic or initially raised and/or on hypoglycaemic drugs.
- Food and fluid intake.

Ⅲ Appendix 4, p.326 is a care pathway directing early monitoring.

Involving therapists

- In a well-organized acute stroke ward, there should be no need for specific referral of patients to therapists by doctors.
- Rehabilitation should start as soon as the patient is able, and this is best assessed daily between therapists and nurses. This may be on day 1.
- Early mobilization is a key feature of specialized stroke unit care.
- Highly successful Scandinavian stroke services describe very aggressive early mobilization even for very severely affected patients (physiotherapist assessment within 6h, out of bed within 24h).
- For less severely affected patients, this will allow early functional mobility or discharge.
- For others, it reduces the chances of venous thrombosis and other complications of immobility. However, it must be safe (avoiding falls, shoulder problems, and injuries to staff), and should not promote abnormal tone, or adversely affect potential for recovery of normal movement patterns.
- Early mobilization is labour intensive. Transferring and standing a hemiplegic patient can take two or more therapists. Mechanical aids (hoists, standing hoists) must be available.
- Physiotherapists will sometimes see unconscious or very ill patients, predominantly to advise on positioning (mainly to improve lung ventilation).
- Occupational therapists' rapid assessment of minimally disabled patients may help early discharge. Otherwise basic assessment can be undertaken if the patient is sufficiently alert, including perceptual and cognitive screening, and ascertaining previous functional and social information.
- Patients with impaired swallowing on initial screening, or communication problems, should be referred to a speech and language therapist, but this can wait a day or two.

Communication

- Good communication is primarily a matter of common courtesy. But adequate explanation may also help reduce anxiety and psychological distress, in both patients and family members. A policy of proactive information giving may reduce complaints.
- Communication may be difficult, because of drowsiness, aphasia, or confusion. Patients often forget what they are told, especially if anxious in the presence of doctors. Explanations may have to be repeated several times.
- Don't assume that all family members get on or share information, although it can be pointed out to them that it helps hard-pressed medical and nursing staff if they can be seen together, or a key-contact person is appointed who will pass on what they are told.
- Patients and their families will need an explanation of:
  - What a stroke is.
  - What the process of care in hospital will be (whether admission is necessary, what follow-up arrangements are if not, where they will be admitted to, what tests or treatment is likely).
  - What the immediate prognosis is (stroke may be life threatening, what good or bad signs there are).
  - When more information will be available.
- Some immediate decision making may be required, that should ideally involve information from, or to, families (e.g. resuscitation).
- Let nursing and medical colleagues know what the diagnosis is, and what your plans are (especially if you are not going to have ongoing responsibility). Best done by writing it clearly in the case notes.

Summary

1. Most patients should be admitted to hospital, unless they are minimally disabled and can be assessed and investigated as an outpatient almost immediately.
2. In hospital, on day 1 you need to make or confirm the diagnosis of stroke, order initial investigations, and instigate plans for relief of pressure areas, feeding, and hydration, maintaining oxygenation, and bladder and bowel management
3. Suitably equipped and trained units should consider thrombolysis for carefully selected patients with ischaemic strokes who arrive at hospital within 3–4h and who can be assessed and treated within an hour (up to 4.5h from onset).
4. Some stroke patients are very ill, and require careful nursing, with particular regard to swallowing, pressure areas, positioning, continence, and care of the unconscious patient.
5. Apart from thrombolysis, initial medical management of cerebral infarcts involves hydration and aspirin. There are likely benefits from a more intensive regimen of physiological monitoring, manipulation of BP to achieve moderate hypertension, and correction in abnormalities in oxygenation, hyperglycaemia, and pyrexia.
6. Supportive management of intracerebral haemorrhage is similar, but antithrombotics must be avoided, anticoagulation or other bleeding disorders reversed, and consideration given to referral to a neurosurgeon for evacuation.
7. Neurological, respiratory, and cardiovascular function, glycaemia, and temperature should be monitored closely over the first 48h at least.
8. Let patients, relatives, and staff colleagues know what has happened and what is planned.

Chapter 3

The first 2 weeks

Trajectories of recovery

We can define four patterns of stroke care (excluding subarachnoid haemorrhage for now):
- TIAs and minor, non-disabling stroke.
- Mildly disabling stroke, which recovers to independence within a week or two.
- Moderate or severe stroke requiring many weeks of rehabilitation to reach maximum abilities.
- Fatal stroke, requiring terminal care.

The objectives are different for each, with some overlap (Table 3.1).
- The first group will often not be admitted to hospital, or should be discharged quickly if they are. Investigation and further management can take place on the day or urgently as an outpatient, but if facilities are not available for this, they should be admitted to a specialist ward.
- The other three groups should be admitted to a specialist ward.
- We will consider terminal care separately (see 📖 Chapter 7, p.157).

Table 3.1 Trajectories of stroke care

Trajectory	Objective	Action
Non-disabling	Information	Explanation and reassurance
	Aetiology	Investigation
	Secondary prevention	Carotid duplex, cardiac rhythm and function, antithrombotics, BP and cholesterol reduction, smoking cessation, lifestyle advice
	Out-patient management	Refer to specialist clinic
Minor disabling	Information	Explanation and reassurance
	Aetiology	Investigation
	Secondary prevention	As for non-disabling stroke
	Functional assessment/ rehabilitation	Nursing, SLT, OT, and physiotherapy
	Rapid discharge	Accessing community rehabilitation and follow-up services
Moderate–severe disabling	Diagnosis	Review by expert clinician
	Survival	Physiological support, nursing care
	Avoidance of complications	Expert nursing and medical care
	Securing hydration and nutrition	Monitor swallowing, IV, nasogastrically, or gastrostomy
	Rehabilitation	Nursing, SLT OT, and physiotherapy on a dedicated ward
Fatal	Diagnosis	Review by expert clinician
	Freedom from distress	Necessary palliative treatment
	Dignity	Avoidance of unnecessary intervention

OT, occupational therapy; SLT, speech and language therapy.

Feeding and hydration

About half of patients admitted to hospital following a stroke cannot swallow safely. Mortality in this group is high, but the majority of survivors regain their swallowing eventually. Of those with problems initially:
- Half are dead by 6 weeks.
- 30% can feed orally within 2 weeks.
- Most of the rest recover safe swallowing over the next month.
- Long-term survival without safe swallowing is quite uncommon.

Hydration is important:
- Thirst is unpleasant, initially at least, in conscious patients before renal failure and drowsiness take over.
- Dehydration and pre-renal renal failure can develop.
- Venous thrombosis and pressure sores are more likely in dehydrated patients.
- Inadequate cardiac filling pressure may result in decreased BP, which may be harmful to the perfusion of the stroke 'penumbra'.
- Death results after 1–2 weeks with no fluid intake.

Nutrition is important:
- Hunger is unpleasant.
- Malnutrition is associated with worse outcomes and a slower rate of recovery.
- Under conditions of subnutrition, muscle is catabolized to meet metabolic needs. Resulting muscular weakness increases disability, which must be reversed during rehabilitation.
- Vitamin deficiencies or insufficiencies can occur (e.g. vitamin K increasing prothrombin time/international normalized ratio (INR), vitamin D causing myopathy and bone demineralization, especially in the face of immobility).
- Prolonged undernutrition suppresses immune function.
- Loss of 20–30% body weight results in depressed mood, which is difficult to reverse until body weight is restored.
- Wound healing (e.g. pressure sores or leg ulcers) is inhibited by poor nutrition.
- Many drugs are best given orally—there may be problems if some are omitted (e.g. for Parkinson's disease or heart failure, or those dependent on benzodiazepines).

A simple premise in clinical nutrition is that 'if there is a functioning gut, use it'. The problem in stroke care is accessing it.

Some guidelines assist safe oral feeding:
- Thickened liquids, and cold, soft, single consistency foods are easier to swallow.
- You cannot swallow with your neck extended. Sit the patient up. Achieving this for someone with very poor trunk control is not easy, and can be labour intensive.
- Risk of aspiration can be reduced by flexing the neck ('a chin tuck') before swallowing (this closes the airway and opens the gullet).
- Pacing—take it slowly, allow time for each mouthful to be cleared before giving another. Some patients 'pouch' food in their cheeks if they cannot swallow it. This needs removing (with a drink or a finger at the end of the meal.

If, despite these measures, swallowing is unsafe by day 2, consider nasogastric feeding. Mouth care and monitoring for recovery of swallowing should continue. A standardized tube-feeding regimen can be used initially. Refer to a dietician for assessment of individualized nutrition requirements and an appropriate feed prescription.

Nasogastric feeding has problems:
- Tubes are uncomfortable, both when inserted and when in place, and are often displaced or pulled out.
- Occasionally they can be misplaced into the trachea, and ensuring that this has not occurred causes much testing, delays, and missed feed or medication. If an acid pH (<5.5) can be detected on pH indicator paper after aspiration of stomach contents from the tube, then the tube is in the stomach. However, often an aspirate cannot be obtained, or is found not to be acidic (due to proton pump inhibitor drugs or age-related achlorhydria). In this case a chest X-ray is needed. Blowing air down the tube with a syringe and auscultating the abdomen as a test for position is unreliable.
- Oesophageal peristalsis is disrupted, and reflux of feed can occur.
- Liquid feeds can cause diarrhoea.
- A loop or bridle passed behind the nasal septum can effectively secure a nasogastric tube, reducing the need for reinsertion and increasing feed volume delivered.

As an alternative, percutaneous endoscopic (PEG) or radiologically-guided gastrostomy (RIG) can be used:
- They cause little discomfort (after the first couple of days), are difficult to dislodge, and can be managed in rehabilitation hospitals, nursing homes, or at home.
- They may suffer fewer problems with reflux than nasogastric tubes.
- The procedure is under local anaesthetic with midazolam sedation. (Removal may require a further endoscopy.)
- If the patient is not fit for endoscopy, or there are other reasons why this is technically difficult, radiological insertion (with ultrasound or fluoroscopy guidance) is possible.
- In the longer term they require some maintenance to prevent embedding in the gastric mucosa. The tube should be loosened, and rotated every 3–4 weeks.

When to consider gastrostomy feeding is difficult. There are no hard clinical benefits from early placement (Box 3.1). We suggest that gastrostomy placement can be deferred until there is a clear need:
- If a nasogastric tube cannot be tolerated or kept in, gastrotomy insertion may be considered early (within a week if need be).
- If it is anticipated that long-term gastrostomy feeding will be required (about 4–6 weeks after onset, in the absence of clear signs that swallow is improving).
- If transfer to a rehabilitation facility that cannot manage a nasogastric tube is contemplated (although such 'system-centred' care is generally to be deprecated).

Box 3.1 Nutritional supplements, timing, and type of tube feeding (FOOD trials)

- Poor nutrition is seen in 8–34% of patients presenting with stroke, may worsen in hospital, and is associated with poorer outcomes.
- Three linked randomized controlled trials used a common design, amongst patients with acute first or recurrent stroke:
  - Normal diet (n= 2007) vs oral protein-calorie supplementation (n= 2016).
  - Early tube feeding (n=429) vs tube feeding avoided for at least 7 days (n=430).
  - Nasogastric (n=159) vs PEG (n= 162) tube feeding.
- The oral supplementation trial was for patients who could swallow safely, and delivered 360mL per day containing 6.3kJ and 63mg protein/mL until discharge (median length of stay 34 days). After 6 months follow-up relative risks with supplements were:
  - 0.94 (95% CI 0.78–1.13) for death (12% vs 13%).
  - 1.03 (95% CI 0.91–1.17) for death or dependency (59% vs 59%).
  - Complications, causes of death, length of stay, and quality of life were similar.
  - There was a trend towards benefit in those initially clinically undernourished (22% reduced risk of death or dependency), and harm in those overweight, but no other subgroups showed differences.
- The early tube feeding trial was for dysphagic patients. After 6 months follow-up relative risks with early tube feeding were:
  - 0.79 (95% CI 0.6–1.03) for death (42% vs 48%).
  - 0.93 (95% CI 0.37–1.3) for death or dependency (79% vs 80%).
  - Therefore, early tube feeding reduced case fatality at the expense of increasing the proportion surviving with a poor outcome.
- The nasogastric vs PEG trial was also for dysphagic patients. After 6 months follow-up relative risks with PEG tube feeding were:
  - 1.04 (95% CI 0.67–1.61) for death (49% vs 48%).
  - 1.86 (0.99–3.5) for death or dependency (89% vs 81%).
- There were no major differences in other outcomes between the early vs avoid groups or the nasogastric vs PEG groups.
- Early tube feeding is unlikely to be hazardous, but differences in outcome were small, and there was an excess of dependent survivors. Data do not support a policy of routine early PEG insertion. Nutritional supplements are probably only beneficial in those initially undernourished.

Lancet 2005; **365**:755–63; 764–72.

The practicalities of insertion are listed in Table 3.2. It takes a few days to think about, discuss, and organize.

Videopharyngography ('videofluoroscopy', an X-ray test of swallowing) may be required where 'silent aspiration' is suspected, usually on the advice of a speech and language therapist.

Table 3.2 Practical issues surrounding gastrostomy tube insertion

Issue	Action
Periprocedure mortality is about 1%	Inform patient and/or family
Desirability	Full information and counselling required
Consent	Formal consent necessary, or best interest assessment if lacking capacity
Clotting (may be deranged after starvation)	Check FBC, INR, and APTT. Give vitamin K if necessary
Dehydration	Check electrolytes and renal function, correct IV if necessary
Respiratory function—dangerous desaturation can occur during endoscopy	Optimize. Postpone if active chest infection. Consider radiological placement
Previous gastric surgery, severe obesity	Consult endoscopist. Consider radiological placement
If prolonged starvation or severe malnutrition, possible refeeding syndrome (electrolyte derangement, rhabdomyolysis, heart and respiratory failure, hypotension, arrhythmias, seizures, coma)	Give thiamine, start feed slowly, monitor serum phosphate, potassium, magnesium, and calcium daily for first 4 days, and correct. If phosphate <0.5mmol/L, give IV phosphate 50mmol over 24h. Repeat if necessary

Neurological problems

Hemiparesis

- Weakness may affect the face, arm, or leg, or a more limited part such as the hand.
- The extent of paralysis may deteriorate in the first week, probably as the ischaemic penumbra infarcts, or a small, deep, end-artery progressively occludes. No proven intervention can avert this (apart from early aspirin, to a small extent). Measures to optimize physiology (BP, oxygenation, blood glucose, temperature) probably help. Anticoagulation does not improve outcome overall (fewer infarcts are offset with an equal number of new intracerebral bleeds). The combination of aspirin and clopidogrel (in the short term) is of uncertain benefit.
- Resistance to passive movement (tone), reflecting resting muscle activity, is often low initially, but may be normal, and can increase over subsequent days or weeks (spasticity may develop).
- Cortical infarcts (TACI and PACI) typically affect the arm more than the leg. This is because the motor cortex supplying the leg derives its blood supply partly from the anterior cerebral artery (rather than the middle cerebral artery).
- Isolated anterior cerebral artery infarcts (the leg is affected and the arm spared) is possible but uncommon—review the diagnosis.
- Subcortical infarcts (lacunar strokes, affecting the internal capsule or brainstem tracts) often result in a dense, flaccid, paralysis of both arm and leg equally.

Recovery of hemiparesis is a combination of three things:
- Spontaneous recovery.
- Active therapy.
- Avoidance of complications.

Spontaneous recovery accounts for the greater part. Increasing evidence suggests that active therapy is important to maximize and make use of the recovery, without developing or reinforcing increased tone and dysfunctional, abnormal movements:
- If paralysis is severe, initial management tries to re-establish head and trunk stability using therapeutic positioning and limb support, to achieve sitting, independence in eating, and upper body self-care.
- Early muscle use stimulates neuroplasticity and normal muscular activation, e.g. sitting and standing help develop trunk control.
- Early standing promotes muscle activation through weight bearing, provides sensory feedback, and improves alertness, pressure area care, bowel function, and morale.
- Early training in functional tasks (e.g. transfers) makes handling easier, and reduces the chances of complications.
- The patient is taught to minimize compensatory tactics and overuse of the unaffected side. This encourages activity on the affected side, and avoids reinforcement of abnormal movement patterns.
- Encourage active use of a weak but functional arm to maintain sensory and proprioceptive input, and minimize muscle atrophy.

- Therapists gradually 'progress' activity and use a teaching approach to promote 'carry over' between sessions. The emphasis is on relearning normal movement patterns that can be built upon.
- These principles must be continued throughout the 24-h period to maximize effect, so nurses must be familiar with the moving and handling plan, in consultation with physiotherapists.

Aphasia (or dysphasia—they mean the same thing)

The experience of aphasia has been compared with (a non-Russian speaker) travelling on the Moscow Metro. You know where you want to go, and may want to ask a fellow traveller where to get off, but you can't make yourself understood. You can see the signs at the stations and hear people talking, but cannot understand what they mean.

There are a dozen or more subtypes of aphasia. They boil down to:
- Problems with expression (expressive).
- Problems with understanding (receptive).
- Both together (mixed).

Relatives (and some non-specialist staff) may think the patient has become confused. They may respond by treating him or her as if they had.
- Doctors, nurses, and therapists should discuss functional communication (expression and understanding).
- Explain repeatedly to the patient, and relatives, the nature of the problem.
- Empathize. Imagine what it would be like if it happened to you (one day in several decades time it may). You would find life frustrating, possibly unbearably so. You probably wouldn't understand what was going on. You would wonder if you were going to recover, but might fear that you would not. Lack of communication ability may lead you to be incontinent, thirsty, or in pain. Cooperation with therapy may be hard, and you might be thought to be difficult or unmotivated.
- Assume that understanding is retained, even when expression is severely affected. Explain that the stroke disconnected the thinking bit of the brain from the speaking bit (or disconnected the hearing bit from the understanding bit). Explain the same to family members.
- Encourage visitors not to give up, give the patient time to get things out, and use language as much as possible with the patient.

What to do:
- Get an early SLT assessment, and advice on non-verbal communication, for both staff and relatives.
- Keep language simple. No long or obscure words. Short sentences. One idea at a time. No double negatives. Avoid medical jargon. It may help to imagine you are talking to a non-native English speaker who has basic but limited English.
- Give plenty of time. Repeat or explain if necessary.
- Use gesture, written words, symbols, or pictures (there are books of commonly useful pictures to help, e.g. *The Aphasia Handbook*: Parr S; Connect Press 2004 and *Stroke Talks*: Cottrell S, Davies A; Connect Press 2006).

- The disorder is of language rather than speaking, so written communication will usually be affected also. In any case, often the patient's writing hand will be affected. But it is worth writing things down to see if it helps.
- It is rare for aphasia to occur in complete isolation. There are often visuospatial problems or apraxia as well, even if there is no hemiparesis. Always get an occupational therapy assessment.

Speech and language therapists are experts in communication and strategies to get round problems. High-intensity therapy targeted at specific aspects of language function improves communication. In addition, therapists have a role in advising on alternative communication strategies, and advising, counselling, and supporting the relatives of people with aphasia.

Occupational therapists use an alternative approach. Practising familiar functional tasks (e.g. washing and dressing) allows engagement, and rehabilitation of trunk and upper limbs without the patient being necessarily able to follow instruction.

Emotional lability or emotionalism
- This is emotional expression (usually crying, sometimes anger, rarely laughing) which is inappropriate to (or extreme for) the emotional context.
- It is not the same as depression, but is disabling and distressing to the patient (and those around them).
- Develops (in 15%) over the first week or two.
- Degrees of severity can be defined by the emotional content of triggers (usually spoken statements) which bring on the crying.
- Examine the mental state further, as depression (major affective disorder) is also a cause of crying.
- Explain the problem to patient and relatives.
- Usually responds within a few days to selective serotonin reuptake inhibitors (SSRIs) (citalopram 20mg od) or tricyclic antidepressants (lofepramine 70mg at night)—quicker than you would expect for depression.
- Tends to resolve or improve over time.

Neglect (Table 3.3)
Unawareness or relative disregard of one side of the world is a feature of parietal lobe damage, typically, but not exclusively, when the non-dominant side is affected. If it occurs with dominant parietal lobe lesions, assessment is often complicated by communication problems. It may be transient or persisting, and lesser degrees are often missed.
- Do not confuse with hemianopia (which may also cause problems with perception on one side, but which is more easily compensated by moving the point of visual fixation).
- Can be a major barrier to rehabilitation and recovery.
- Needs looking for explicitly. Doctors, nurses, and therapists may all help in recognizing it.
- Pencil and paper tests, more formal 'parietal lobe batteries' or neuropsychological assessment can be used. Tests include Albert's test (line cancellation), star cancellation, clock face drawing, or drawing double-headed flowers.

- Spontaneous recovery is more important than specific therapy, but patients can be taught to scan to the affected side, if they are able to remember.
- Reduce isolation by positioning (with respect to walls, etc.) so that the non-neglected side is facing the world. An older fashion for 'forcing' use of the neglectful side by doing the converse was not helpful.
- Explain it to relatives—as with all bizarre and unusual phenomena.

Table 3.3 Aspects of neglect

Feature	Description
Visual extinction	Failure to register a stimulus such as finger movement in the periphery of a visual field, when a similar, simultaneous, stimulus is applied to the opposite side
Sensory extinction	Failure to register a tactile stimulus such as hand touching, when a similar, simultaneous, stimulus is applied to the opposite side
Topographical neglect	Neglect during drawing, copying, constructional tasks, line cancellation or bisection
Hemi-inattention	Behaviour during clinical examination or therapy suggesting inability to respond to environmental stimuli on one side (noises, people approaching)
Anosognosia	Denial of the presence of neurological deficit such as weakness. Can result in falls and fractures if the patient confidently tries to walk on a paralysed leg
Denial of body parts	Denial of ownership, lack of awareness of a limb
Anosodiasphoria	Lack of concern for the neurological deficit

Other features of parietal lobe dysfunction

- Agnosia—inability to recognize objects.
- Astereognosis—inability to recognize objects placed in the affected hand.
- Agraphaesthesia—inability to recognize a number drawn (with the examiner's finger) on the palm of the patient's hand.
- Geographical disorientation—inability to navigate, or gets lost in, familiar surroundings, despite the ability to see.
- Dressing apraxia—inability to dress (or perform other purposeful constructional tasks) in the absence of weakness, sensory or visual loss, or neglect that would explain it. May occur in a pure form.

Pain

Pain is cited as a problem with remarkable frequency after stroke, which many doctors find surprising. Pain divides between stroke-specific pain (central poststroke pain, CPSP; shoulder pain) and comorbid pain, which is common in the older population anyway, but which may be exacerbated by stroke (e.g. back or knee pain, associated with poor positioning or muscular deconditioning).

CPSP is difficult to assess and manage. It often has a vague or ill-defined quality to it, both in the symptom and its localization. Some patients are reluctant to call it 'pain', rather than an annoying or unpleasant feeling. It is confined to the affected side, and may have an aching or burning quality, possibly with hyperaesthesia or allodynia (unpleasant sensation of normal tactile stimuli). Depression and anxiety may exacerbate. Simple analgesia is rarely helpful, and low-dose amitriptyline (25–100mg od) alone often disappointing. Pregabalin (50–100mg bd, alone or added to amitriptyline) is probably the most effective drug, but even this does not always work, and may be limited by side effects. Tramadol, other opiates, acupuncture, or TENS (transcutaneous electrical nerve stimulation) sometimes help. The goal of treatment may be to make the pain less distressing, rather than to cure it completely.

Other pains may also be distressing, and a barrier to regaining function. There may be several different pains; each needs assessing and treating or palliating. Always reassess drug treatments for effect, optimal dose, and side effects. Other professional disciplines, especially physiotherapists, may also be able to help, and clinical psychologists may try a cognitive behavioural approach.

Shoulder pain tends to become a problem later (and persist). It is discussed on p.200 and p.201).

Persisting drowsiness

Most patients who are initially drowsy either die or recover in the first week or two. A few patients who remain drowsy are especially problematic. They are not fit enough to engage in therapy, and appear to be in 'limbo':

- Exclude metabolic, infective, and drug causes.
- Consider hydrocephalus and recurrent stroke—repeat the CT scan.
- The patient may be terminally ill, and a decision to withdraw active or supportive treatments may need to be taken.
- Some patients have prolonged periods of drowsiness or sleeping, and be fairly well during the few hours they are awake. Modafinil (100mg od increasing up to bd, morning and noon, or 200mg bd), or dexamphetamine (5mg od, increasing every few days up to 60mg/day) can be tried. Watch for hypertension and fits.

Neurological deterioration

A common reason for requesting a medical review is because of neuro-logical deterioration (Table 3.4). It may occur at any time. This may be:
- Decreased level of consciousness.
- Fitting.
- Worsening focal neurological signs.

Transtentorial herniation is the commonest cause of death in the first week. It generally:
- Occurs within 24h of bleeds.
- Peaks at days 4–5 after infarction (due to oedema formation).

Haemorrhagic transformation occurs in 75% of cardioembolic strokes, and 30% of all infarcts, within 4 days. Neurological deterioration occurs in 20% of these.

Table 3.4 Neurological deterioration after stroke

Cause	Action
'Evolving' stroke—worsening initial symptoms over 24h or so	Review diagnosis, early CT scan. Anticoagulation is not indicated
Raised intracranial pressure (oedema), herniation, hydrocephalus	Repeat CT scan. In the UK, mostly just observation. Consider mannitol or neurosurgical opinion
Recurrent stroke	Seek 'active' embolic source (e.g. cardiac, including endocarditis), alternative diagnosis, e.g. vasculitis or fits. Otherwise manage as first stroke
Haemorrhagic transformation of infarct	Stop aspirin or anticoagulants
Intercurrent infection	Check white cell count and inflammatory markers, review especially chest and urine
Drug adverse effect	Review
Metabolic disturbance	Check glucose, electrolytes (syndrome of inappropriate secretion of antidiuretic hormone [SIADH] in 10% of strokes)
Fitting (about 5% in acute phase)	Clinical diagnosis, need eye witness account. Likely to recur if after the first 24h. Oral sodium valproate is antiepileptic drug of choice, or IV phenytoin if no oral access

Medical problems

Hypertension

- BP goes up after a stroke, and comes down again over the next week.
- Initial BP is related to outcome (fatality is least in those with initial systolic pressures of 140–180mmHg), but it is unclear if any manipulations, up or down, improve outcomes.
- Unless there is evidence of immediate end-organ damage (encephalopathy, heart or renal failure) or other hypertensive emergency (see Chapter 2, p.31), do not give antihypertensive drugs for at least a week.
- As far as we know at present, BP reduction is primarily a longer-term (months to years) secondary preventative intervention, so there is no hurry.
- However, it is logistically convenient to establish a secondary prevention regimen whilst the patient is in hospital.
- After the first week, the ward BP record makes a good assessment of 'usual' BP.
- Start with bendroflumethazide 2.5mg od, and add a calcium channel blocker (amlodipine 5–10mg od) or an angiotensin-converting enzyme inhibitor (ACEI; any will do, e.g. ramipril 5–10mg od, or lisinopril 5–40 mg od), unless there are strong contraindications, or indications for using something else. See Chapter 10, p.233.

Hyperglycaemia

- If glucose is raised initially, it will often also come down of its own accord over a few days (a 'stress' response).
- There is observational evidence (cohort studies) that initially raised glucose is associated with poorer outcomes. The single trial to address the issue therapeutically was underpowered, and neither demonstrated nor excluded worthwhile benefit (Box 2.5).
- Raised glucose can be reduced (insulin sliding scale) to keep the blood sugar at 4–10mmol/L. This is labour intensive, and needs a lot of finger-prick monitoring, so should be converted rapidly to a twice-daily insulin regimen (isophane or isophane/soluble mix).
- If requirements are low, and oral feeding has been re-established, try withdrawing therapy, or converting to oral hypoglycaemics after a week.
- Remember the longer-term objectives of diabetes management:
  - Avoidance of symptoms (thirst, polyuria, pruritis).
  - Avoidance of diabetic crises (hypoglycaemia, ketoacidosis and non-ketotic hyperosmolar coma)
  - Avoidance of (micro-) vascular complications in the longer term.
- The newly diagnosed diabetic will need a strategic plan. The symptoms most likely to cause problems are polyuria and nocturia—especially if the stroke has left the bladder unstable and mobility uncertain. Hypoglycaemia is more likely to be a problem than hyperglycaemic states if elderly or frail. Moderately tight control should be the goal—pre-meal blood glucose measurements of 5–12mmol/L.

- Maintaining euglycaemia is an ineffective way of avoiding macrovascular complications. The full range of alternative vascular preventative measures is required.
- Diabetic complications may complicate rehabilitation, including retinopathy and cataract, peripheral vascular disease, peripheral neuropathy (compromises balance), and neuropathic and ischaemic foot ulcers.

An admission for stroke is an opportunity to ensure that comprehensive screening for diabetic complications is performed (dilated fundoscopy, renal function and proteinuria, test foot sensation, foot care).

Medical complications

A 'complication' is a secondary disease or condition aggravating a previous one. Stroke care is medically active—50% or more of patients develop medical complications. Risk of complications increases with stroke severity, and is greatest in the first week.

It is useful to distinguish between:
- Neurological features of the initial stroke, such as spasticity, dysphagia, neglect, or fitting.
- Effects of recurrent stroke, or other coincidental vascular events (e.g. heart attack).
- Effects of pre-existing, comorbid, conditions (e.g. arthritis, dementia).
- 'True' complications—new conditions arising because of the stroke.
- Associated medical conditions—such as high BP, hyperglycaemia.

All of these increase the complexity of managing stroke. Each problem needs to be managed carefully and optimally, to ensure the best chance of a good outcome.

'True complications' are dominated by the effects of immobility, and psychological responses (Table 3.5).

Chest infections result from aspiration, drowsiness, and immobility. Urinary infections are usually catheter associated, but are common in elderly women in any case.

DVTs:
- Develop in 50% of patients with a hemiplegia, but are usually subclinical.
- Clinically apparent DVT occurs in about 5%.
- Clinically important pulmonary emboli occur in 1–2 %, but are common at postmortem amongst patients who die after 2–4 weeks.
- Early LMWH or anticoagulation prevents DVT, but appears to have little impact on overall outcome.
- Aspirin is also an effective venous antithrombotic, but full-length compression stockings are ineffective.

Table 3.5 True complications of stroke

Problem	Action
Infections	Care over feeding. Avoid urinary catheters if possible. Monitor carefully to diagnose early
Venous thrombo-embolism	Hydration, early mobilization, aspirin. Prophylactic LMWH if high risk. Anticoagulant dose LMWH and warfarin for proven thromboses (or a caval filter if an intracerebral bleed)
Pressure sores	Early assessment, pressure relieving mattress, and turning regimen. Early mobilization
Joint contractures	Positioning, early physiotherapy, thermoplastic splinting, botulinum toxin
Osteoporosis	Vitamin D supplementation may help prevent. Bisphosphonate if history of low trauma fracture (see 📖 Falls and fractures, p 312)
Depression and anxiety	Positive therapeutic environment. Problem solving. Communication, sympathetic staff. May require antidepressant drugs, but do not rush in
Falls and fractures	Moving and handling assessment by nurses, physiotherapists, and occupational therapists. Suitable walking aids, adequate supervision. Appropriate footwear. Minimize sedative medication. Test for postural hypotension. Bedrails (cotsides) may help or may hinder. Consider hip protectors
Paresis or dependent oedema	Elevation (lying down, rather than footstool). Compression stockings or pneumatic boots (Flowtron). Diuretics in severe cases (furosemide 20–40mg od)
Shoulder pain or subluxation	Do not pull shoulder, or lift under arm. Careful positioning in bed and when sitting in chair. Adequate support. Physiotherapy advice. Occupational therapists assess for specialist mechanical supports. Simple analgesics, consider steroid injection or suprascapular nerve block

Bladder and bowel management

Incontinence of one or both of urine and faeces is unpleasant and distressing.

- Urinary incontinence:
  - Is predominantly detrusor instability. This recovers at the same rate as other neurological functions.
  - A proportion have incomplete bladder emptying, either caused by the stroke, or a comorbidity.
  - A further proportion (perhaps a quarter) have normal bladders, but cannot communicate or move well enough to get to a toilet or urinal in time.
- Before acting, have some idea of what the diagnosis is:
  - Exclude infection (dipstick, specimen for culture, if possible).
  - Exclude retention (portable bladder ultrasound scanner).
  - Record a 48-h urine output (frequency–volume) chart.
- If the patient is aphasic, has other communication problems, or dementia, offer the toilet at least every 2h (they may have bladder instability as well).
- Anticholinergic medication is relatively ineffective, and prone to side effects, so should be reserved until the acute phase is over, and coa-operation with a prompted voiding regimen or bladder retraining is possible.
- Sometimes a catheter will be requested. If a patient can possibly be managed using incontinence pads or a sheath catheter, these should be tried. Catheters always have problems (bladder spasm with by-passing, infection, blockage, urethral trauma). In one stroke unit trial, the patients on the unit had half the number of urinary infections of those on general medical wards—neatly matched by the prevalence of catheter usage.
- Use an indwelling catheter only if there is a good reason e.g. a patient who is developing sore skin, or with incomplete bladder emptying who is difficult to catheterize or who finds intermittent catheterization distressing. Reassess the need for it regularly. Anticholinergic drugs (e.g. trospium 20mg bd or tolterodine MR 4mg od) can be used for catheter-induced bladder spasm.
- A care pathway is given on 📖 Appendix 10, p.340. See also 📖 Chapter 8, p.202.

Managing faecal incontinence in acute stroke is difficult. Make sure the following are not responsible:

- Laxatives or other drugs.
- Acute diarrhoeal diseases (infections, inflammatory bowel disease).
- Tube feeds.
- Communication problems.
- Access to toilets, commode, or bedpan.
- Constipation.

Do a rectal examination to exclude impaction. An abdominal X-ray can help, if feasible. An immobile, dehydrated, or undernourished person is at high risk of constipation. Primarily a stimulant laxative is required (i.e. senna—use an adequate dose, up to 30mg or 4 tablets, or 20mL syrup per day). If tube fed, fibre-added feeds can help. Sodium docusate (200mg bd) is a 'wetting agent', and acts as both a softener and stimulant, and is a useful adjunct to senna. Osmotic laxatives are sometimes required in addition.

Other mechanisms include:
• Lack of awareness.
• Colorectal disinhibition,

In these cases, formal bowel regimens may be useful in the longer term (see 🕮 p.204), but have no place in the acute phase. Containment in pads, which are changed rapidly if soiled, is probably the best option. Faecal containment bags, sometimes used on intensive care units, are a little-used alternative.

Continue to assess over time, and review for opportunities to intervene.

Starting rehabilitation

There is no clear cut-point between acute and rehabilitation phases:
- If the patient is well enough, therapy should start immediately.
- Therapy should be as intensive as possible—the maximum tolerated daily, although this is may be constrained by patient fatigue or staff availability.

Physiotherapy

- Physiotherapists should be involved early, and should make their own assessment of how much they can work with a patient.
- Early mobilization is associated with better outcomes—even after taking account of the potential confounding influence of disease severity (the least badly affected can mobilize sooner, and do better, quite apart from their early mobility).
- If rehabilitation is to take place on a different ward from acute care, the care received should be made as seamless as possible. Type and intensity of therapy should be determined by the patient's needs not location.

Mobility-related work in less severely affected patients will be undertaken by nurses and occupational therapists as well as physiotherapists:
- They should make their own judgements about what is safe and desirable to do, but must have ready access to a physiotherapist in contentious or difficult cases.
- Delaying mobilization pending a physiotherapist's assessment indicates a poorly staffed or poorly organized system.

Occupational therapy

Early occupational therapy intervention is beneficial. Initial tasks involve:
- Assessment and information gathering, including for neglect, apraxias, and cognitive problems, which can be difficult to detect, and may have a bearing on subsequent functional tasks.
- Work on practically-focused tasks such as dressing, are important morale boosters, as well as being important for discharge planning.
- Work on upper body personal care contributes to improved trunk control in patients with a severe hemiparesis.

Many day-to-day functional activities will be managed by nurses, so there must be good communication between them and other therapists. This involves:
- Understanding by nurses of what is possible and desirable in the view of therapists.
- Trust in nurses' judgement, and avoidance of overprotectiveness.
- It is possible that rehabilitation nursing, rather than any other type of therapy, makes the major difference between specialized stroke units and management on general wards.

Speech and language therapy

- Speech and language therapists spend much of their time with acute stroke patients dealing with swallowing problems.
- A careful interface with nursing judgement is required. Starving a patient whilst awaiting a speech therapy assessment may not be necessary if *suitably trained* or experienced nurses can use their judgement in trying thickened fluids and soft foods.
- Communication assessment should not be neglected. The sudden onset of aphasia is a distressing and bewildering experience for both patients and carers, which can make discharge from hospital difficult.

Documenting changes and progress

Communication is always important when a diverse group of professionals are working with a given patient.

If staff responsible for a patient change frequently, they are unlikely to get to grips with problems, cannot establish a rapport with patients or families, and may miss things. Good case notes are necessary to communicating progress, problems, and plans.

Information is required on:
- Progress of neurological impairments.
- Progress in aetiological investigation.
- Medical complications (and the evidence for them) and comorbidities.
- Discussions with the patient and family.
- Documentation of decisions made.
- Functional ability.
- Home circumstances, family or other support, prospects, and progress towards discharge.

Multidisciplinary notes are sometimes used. A weekly (or more frequent) team meeting should be convened and thoroughly documented:
- Physiotherapists will often have the best day-to-day news on motor impairments.
- Occupational therapists may help in the assessment of neglect and apraxias, and will start collecting information about the home environment and support.
- Speech and language therapists may report on progress with communication and swallowing.
- Nurses will know best about day-to-day functional performance.
- Problems emerging in functional tasks may prompt medical review (pain, breathlessness, dizziness, depression).

Any of these may collect information about pre-morbid abilities and home circumstances. In this case, demarcation between professions is not clear cut. Share information and avoid duplication if possible (if nothing else, it undermines the confidence of patients and carers to be asked the same information three or four times).

Moving on

What happens after the acute ward depends on how services are configured in any one place:
- Some services combine acute and rehabilitation care.
- Some separate them out.
- Some combine stroke and generic rehabilitation.
- Others specialize.
- Some have well-developed home rehabilitation.

There is no clear-cut point when acute care becomes rehabilitation. Involvement of rehabilitation therapists is beneficial at an early stage. Continuity may be best served by keeping all stroke care in one place.

On the other hand, acute care and rehabilitation sometimes sit uncomfortably together. If you are worrying about drips and measuring blood glucose, you are less likely to walk the patient to the toilet, talk about fears and thwarted ambitions, or make plans for going home.

Size of service and availability of beds is also important. A large service can justify separate wards better than a small one. And rehabilitation may, of necessity, take place on an acute ward, whilst a place on a rehabilitation ward is awaited.

There are two important questions that need answering at this point:
- Can the patient go home?
- Should the patient move to a specialist rehabilitation ward?

Going home

We will discuss discharge planning, and options for home rehabilitation, later (see 📖 Chapter 9, p.219). 'Can this patient go home?' must be asked an early stage. For this to succeed:
- The patient must be medically stable (i.e. neurologically stable, free from debilitating infection, severe metabolic disturbance, or cardio-respiratory problems such as hypotension, unstable cardiac rhythms, untreated heart or respiratory failure, acute coronary syndromes).
- Able to feed and maintain hydration adequately.
- As a minimum, be able to transfer to the commode by day and at night, alone or with a willing carer.
- Plans made for pressure area relief.
- Plans made for managing continence problems.
- Plans made for delivering medication.
- Plans made for continuing rehabilitation, if required, at home, in a day hospital or as an outpatient.

If 'returning home' means returning to a residential or nursing home, be aware of the difference between them:
- A residential home provides 'board, lodging, and personal care'. Although criteria vary, they cannot as a rule cope with severely disabled or ill patients.
- Nursing homes have at least one registered nurse on duty all the time, and they can cope with much more severe levels of disability. But they are not hospitals. If and when to discharge is a matter for negotiation between the patient, the home and your (team's) assessment of how well the setting can provide for any ongoing rehabilitation needs.

Transfer to a rehabilitation ward

Rehabilitation wards vary. Some take patients early, and manage 'acute' problems such as dysphagia. Some provide very intensive rehabilitation. They may require patients to be:

- Fully alert.
- Cognitively able to follow instructions and retain ('carry over') what is learnt.
- Robust enough to take part in rehabilitation without tiring unduly.
- Free from major comorbidity.

Given the nature of the population, however, the system must also include wards which will take on as many problems as the patient presents. These include cognitive impairment, multiple comorbidities, and lack of stamina. However, a designated rehabilitation ward, which may be off the acute general hospital site, could reasonably expect a patient to be:

- Medically stable.
- Free from infectious diarrhoea (including *Clostridium difficile*—although methicillin-resistant *Staphylococcus aureus* [MRSA] colonization is not necessarily a bar to management on a rehabilitation ward).
- Able to swallow safely, and maintain adequate nutrition (or have a PEG tube sited).
- Not imminently awaiting tests or opinions, such as CT scans, necessitating an unpleasant ambulance journey back to the acute hospital, and possibly tying up a member of staff for a morning.

There is no evidence to suggest that those with more severe stroke benefit less from active attempts at rehabilitation in specialized units (Box 3.2).

Box 3.2 Stroke unit care is beneficial to patients who have suffered a severe stroke

- 71 patients with severe stroke (selected by initial neurological features, the Orpington Prognostic Score) were randomized between a stroke unit and general ward management.
- Mortality was 21% (stroke unit) vs 46% (general wards).
- Home discharge rate was 47% (stroke unit) vs 21% (general ward).
- Median length of hospital stay was 43 days (stroke unit) vs 59 days (general ward).

Stroke 1995; **26**:2031–4.

What do specialist services do differently?

Specialist services improve outcomes (Box 3.3). The exact reasons are uncertain, but some combination of (multiprofessional) expertise, thoroughness, continuity, and enthusiasm for managing stroke patients clearly makes a difference (Boxes 3.4 and 3.5).

Box 3.3 Improved outcomes with specialist stroke unit management

- Between the 1970s and 2000, 23 randomized controlled trials compared management in geographically-defined stroke units with general medical wards.
- Stroke units varied greatly. Predominantly they were rehabilitation units, some were acute wards, others were mixed.
- Relative risks for stroke unit over general ward care were:
  - 0.80 (95% CI 0.60–1.0) for all-cause mortality.
  - 0.68 (95% CI 0.52–0.84) for combined death or dependency.
- There were no differences in benefits according to age, sex, stroke severity, type of medical department providing the service, timing of admission, or maximum duration of stay.
- Mean length of stay on the stroke units varied from 13 to 162 days, which was in some cases shorter, and others longer, than for the control group. Overall there was little difference.
- There was no clear benefit for dedicated stroke wards over mixed rehabilitation wards (odds ratio for death plus dependency 1.01, 95% CI 0.51–1.51).
- Characteristics of stroke units differing from general wards were coordinated multidisciplinary management, involvement of family in rehabilitation, specialization, and education of staff patients and carers (features you would expect on any good rehabilitation ward).
- Stroke outcomes are sensitive to differences in process, but the most important individual elements remain uncertain.

British Medical Journal 1997; **314**:1151–9; *The Cochrane Library* 2004; Issue 2.

Box 3.4 Possible explanations for better outcomes on stroke units

- Amount, type, or content of remedial therapy.
- Continuity (nurses adopting therapy principles, routines, policies).
- Better identification of stroke-associated impairments and disabilities.
- Assessment and management of comorbidity.
- Prevention, identification, and management of complications.
- Aids, appliances, orthoses, and seating.
- Less competition for medical and nursing time.

- Improved motivation, morale, and psychological support.
- Increased self-directed therapy.
- Communication, education, and involvement of relatives.
- Realistic goal setting and prognostication.
- Discharge planning.
- Follow-up and outreach for late complications.

Box 3.5 How specialist services are different in practice

- An observational study, embedded in a randomized controlled trial (see 📖 Box 2.1, p.35) identified differences in care between a stroke unit and general wards receiving advice from stroke specialists.
- The stroke unit had guidelines for diagnosis, imaging, monitoring (BP, oxygen saturation, blood glucose, fluids and electrolytes, nutrition), and prevention of complications (positioning, swallow assessment, infections, venous thrombosis). Management was multidisciplinary, with early mobilization, individualized rehabilitation plans, and active patient participation.
- The general wards had a peripatetic specialist stroke team, who confirmed the diagnosis and made medical, therapy, and nursing plans, which were implemented by ward staff. The team reviewed patients, set goals, planned treatment and discharge, and liaised with relatives.
- Most aspects of care were comparable, and some differences quite small. However, stroke unit patients were:
  - More thoroughly assessed and monitored for neurological status.
  - More often given oxygen, paracetamol for pyrexia, anticoagulated for AF, screened for swallowing problems, fed early (oral, nasogastric, or PEG in first 7 days).
  - Assessed earlier by occupational therapist and social worker.
  - More often given rehabilitation goals, including higher level tasks and carer needs.
  - Given better secondary prevention.
  - Given more information (as were carers).
- Stroke progression, chest and other infections, dehydration, pressure sores, injurious falls, and other complications were less common on the stroke unit.
- Good outcomes were associated with measures to prevent aspiration, early feeding, and lack of stroke progression, chest infection, and dehydration, but not euglycaemia, or use of oxygen or antipyretics, in a multivariate analysis.
- Even after taking these into account, stroke unit management remained associated with better outcomes, suggesting that other undefined factors were also important.

Lancet 2001; **358**:1586–92.

Summary

1. During the first 2 weeks, some patients die, others recover completely. Some are left with minor disability, with the prospect of rapid rehabilitation and discharge home. Others remain medically and neurologically unstable, and if they survive, have major disability and may need prolonged rehabilitation.

2. If swallowing is unsafe 2 days after the stroke, consider passing a nasogastric tube. If the problem persists beyond 5 or 6 weeks, consider a gastrostomy (remembering these take a few days to organize). Involve a speech and language therapist.

3. Medical complications and neurological deterioration should prompt thorough medical review, to ascertain the diagnosis and institute appropriate management.

4. Bladder and bowel management in the acute phase centres around excluding easily reversible causes, and then adequate containment until the patient is well enough to consider other options.

5. Make early referrals to physiotherapy and occupational therapists.

6. Case notes should be thorough and systematic, recording information from both the medical and functional perspectives. Multidisciplinary team communication should be regular, and well documented.

7. When medically stable and able to maintain nutrition, the patient, may move on to either home rehabilitation or a rehabilitation ward, depending on local services.

Subarachnoid haemorrhage

Subarachnoid haemorrhage (SAH) may initially look like a stroke, but behaves differently. Specialist management is the province of the neurosurgeon, but general and stroke physicians need some grounding in its diagnosis and management.

Incidence is about one-tenth that of other strokes: 10–15 per 100 000 per year. Half present between the ages of 40–55 years. A third occur during sleep, a third during strenuous activity or lifting, and a third during other daytime activities.

What it is

The intracranial vessels lie in the subarachnoid space giving off branches to the brain. Primary SAH occurs when an artery ruptures and blood enters the subarachnoid space. Secondary SAH is extension from a primary intracerebral haemorrhage, or from trauma.

Causes of primary SAH include:
- Ruptured arterial aneurysms (85% of cases, excluding trauma).
- Perimesencephalic SAH (around the brain stem, of uncertain origin, probably venous, 10%).
- Ruptured AVM.
- Rarer causes:
  - Bleeding disorders (including thrombocytopenia, leukaemias).
  - Anticoagulant therapy.
  - Bleeding from tumours.
  - Mycotic aneurysms from endocarditis.
  - Vertebral arterial dissection.
  - Cocaine abuse.
  - Vasculitis.

Blood in the subarachnoid space raises intracranial pressure, irritates the meninges, and causes vasospasm. This produces headache, neck stiffness, risk of coning, and secondary ischaemic brain damage.

Clinical presentation

- Headache, unusually severe, with abrupt (seconds) onset, often described as 'being hit on the back of the head' or an explosion. This may be preceded (in 25%) by a few milder attacks of headache or 'warning leaks'.
- Headache onset may be slower (minutes) in perimesencephalic SAH. Loss of consciousness and focal neurology do not occur.
- You cannot rule out SAH clinically in a patient with sudden-onset headache lasting >2h, even if there are no other symptoms or signs. 25% of sudden-onset headaches are due to SAH, half this if there are no other features. You must get a CT scan, and consider a lumbar puncture.
- Loss of consciousness may follow the headache (in 50%, but it may be brief). Half never wake up. Others are drowsy but not unconscious. Onset may be with a fit (10%).
- Some are confused and irritable (delirious), some vomit at onset, some develop photophobia.
- Signs of meningism develop 3–12h after onset—neck stiffness and Kernig's sign (resistance to knee extension with the hip flexed).
- Some patients also develop early focal neurological signs such as hemiplegia or cranial nerve palsies due to pressure from blood clot or aneurysm, or raised intracranial pressure.
- Blood pressure is high in 50% (some pre-existing, most reactive to the raised intracranial pressure).
- Pyrexia, not due to infection, is common, and may persist for several days. It is associated with poorer outcomes. Half of pyrexial patients have pneumonia, however.
- Examination of the optic fundus may show papilloedema, subhyaloid haemorrhage (in 20%), or vitreous haemorrhage.
- Tendon reflexes may be depressed and plantar responses upgoing.
- An enlarging aneurysm can compress cranial nerves, which may precede rupture (by hours to days):
  - Internal carotid or anterior communicating artery: optic nerve or chiasm—retro-orbital pain and unilateral visual loss.
  - Internal carotid cavernous sinus wall
    - oculomotor (III) nerve: palsy (± Horner's)
    - trochlear (IV) nerve: palsy
    - ophthalmic division of the trigeminal (V) nerve: pain
    - abducens (VI) nerve: palsy.
  - Posterior communicating or basilar artery—retro-orbital pain, and oculomotor (III) palsy.
  - IIIrd and VIth nerve palsy can also indicate tentorial herniation.

Diagnosis

- CT head scan. Confirms the diagnosis in at least 95% of cases, if the scan is done within 48h. Sensitivity is only 50% after a week's delay.
- When the scan is positive, the blood may be:
  - Widespread in the basal cisterns and interhemispheric fissure.
  - Intraventricular (a fluid level in the posterior part of the lateral ventricle).
  - Localized to the site of the ruptured aneurysm, such as the Sylvian fissure from MCA, or interhemispheric fissure due to ruptured anterior communicating artery.
  - Free blood over the cortical sulci.
  - Perimesencephalic haemorrhage—seen in 10%, not usually associated with aneurysms. Blood is around the midbrain in the interpeduncular fossa or localized with no extension to the brain or ventricular systems.
  - In addition there may be:
    - hydrocephalus
    - intracerebral haemorrhage
    - tumour
    - AVMs.
- Lumbar puncture. If the history is suggestive, and CT scan is negative, do a lumbar puncture:
  - To make the diagnosis and rule out meningitis, provided >12h has elapsed from the onset of the headache.
  - Do not do a lumbar puncture if the patient has unreversed anticoagulation (INR >1.5) or thrombocytopenia (platelets <50 × 10⁹/L), or if a supratentorial mass lesion has not been excluded.
  - Negative in 10–15% of SAH.
- Red blood cells appear in CSF as early as 2h after onset, and remain present for 2–3 days. They can also contaminate CSF after a traumatic tap. 12h after SAH, however, the CSF becomes yellow (xanthochromia), and this can be detected spectrophotometrically. It persists for 2 weeks (so can be used to investigate patients who present late after onset of headache). There is also a slightly raised protein and monocytosis.
- Angiography shows an aneurysm in 85%. 10% have more than one aneurysm. Choice of MRA (90% sensitive), CTA, or conventional catheter angiography depends on local availability and expertise.

'Grading' of subarachnoid haemorrhage

The World Federation of Neurological Surgery (WFNS) grades SAHs according to the presenting features (Table 4.1), which guides intervention and prognosis.

Remember that you must diagnose the cause of depressed consciousness. Acute hydrocephalus (progressive drowsiness over first few hours), and comorbid metabolic disorders, are treatable.

There are other prognostic grading systems, so be careful about which one is being referred to.

Table 4.1 World Federation of Neurological Surgery grades for SAH (data from *Journal of Neurosurgery* 1988; **68**:985–6)

Grade	GCS	Focal deficits
I	15	Absent
II	13–14	Absent
III	13–14	Present
IV	7–12	Present or absent
V	3–6	Present or absent

Initial management

- Manage on a high-dependency, critical care, or neurosurgical ward.
- Bed rest until the aneurysm is clipped or coiled.
- Monitor the GCS. Deterioration can mean rebleeding, ischaemia, hydrocephalus, or systemic medical complications.
- Pass a nasogastric tube unless swallowing safely.
- Give paracetamol (1g qds PO or PR) or codeine (30–60mg qds PO, nasogastric tube, or SC) for headache. Avoid sedative drugs.
- Give a stool softener (sodium docusate 200mg bd).
- Give IV saline 3L/day (in addition to enteral intake, giving a total intake up to 6L/day), to prevent hypovolaemia and hyponatraemia due to 'cerebral salt wasting'.
- Monitor fluid balance, measure urea and electrolytes daily.
- Give nimodipine 60mg every 4h PO or nasogastric tube for 21 days, so long as systolic BP is >100mmHg (reduces risk of delayed cerebral ischaemia and poor outcomes—Box 4.1).
- Apart from oral nimodipine do not generally try to lower BP. Any reduction in rebleeding is offset by increased risk of ischaemia. Previous antihypertensive drugs can be continued if the BP is not too low (>140mmHg systolic)
- Liaise early with a neurosurgeon (and/or neuroradiologist) about the strategy for imaging and possible operative intervention. The patient will usually need to be transferred to a neurosurgical centre.
- If there is an associated intraparenchymal haematoma (30% of cases), and progressive decrease in level of consciousness (over the first 2 days) immediate surgical evacuation should be considered. This may prevent herniation.
- Progressive reduction in level of consciousness (possibly with sluggish pupillary responses to light and downward deviation of the eyes), over a few hours, may be due to acute hydrocephalus. Confirm with CT head scan, and refer to a neurosurgeon.

Box 4.1 Trial of nimodipine in SAH

- 554 patients with proven SAH, admitted within 96h, were randomized to 21 days of oral (or nasogastric) nimodipine 60mg 4-hourly or placebo.
- Patients who had SAH producing coma within the week prior to the index event were excluded, otherwise exclusion criteria were minimal.
- 77% of patients had an aneurysm at angiography.
- Relative risks on treatment were:
  - 0.66 (95% CI 0.50–0.87) for cerebral infarction (33% vs 22%).
  - 0.60 (95% CI 0.45–0.80) for death or severe disability (33% vs 20%).
  - 0.71 (95% CI 0.50–1.01) for death (22% vs 15%).
  - 0.65 (95% CI 0.41–1.05) for rebleeding (9% vs 4%).
- Effect of treatment was independent of prognostic factors (including loss of consciousness at onset, age, time to entry, focal neurological signs, and CT and angiographic findings).
- Results were supported in a subsequent meta-analysis, but not where nimodipine was given IV.

British Medical Journal 1989; **298**:636–42.

Selection for imaging and surgery

- Patients in 'good grades' (conscious and without focal neurological signs), and who would be willing to have surgery, should have early angiography.
- If the first angiogram is negative it should be repeated a few days later, unless the bleeding pattern on CT is perimesencephalic.
- If the aneurysm is appropriate, it should be endovascularly coiled (by an interventional neuroradiologist) if there is local expertise (Box 4.2).
- The alternative is surgical clipping, performed within 3 days of initial bleed or after 12 days.
- Early surgery may prevent rebleeds, and reduce delayed ischaemia, but overall there are no clear differences in outcomes between early and late surgery.

Box 4.2 Endovascular coiling or neurosurgical clipping for ruptured aneurysms (International Subarachnoid Aneurysm Trial—ISAT)

- 2143 patients with ruptured intracranial aneurysms randomized to neurosurgical clipping or endovascular coiling (when the aneurysm was technically suitable for either treatment—22% of patients presenting).
- Mean age was 52 years, range 18–87, 88% were WFNS grade 1 or 2. Most were small anterior circulation aneurysms. (Coiling is preferred anyway for posterior circulation aneurysms because of surgical risk, and surgery is generally preferred for MCA aneurysms).
- About 5% of patients allocated to coiling required neurosurgery.
- Relative risks for coiling compared with surgery, at 12 months, were:
  - 0.88 (95% CI 0.73–1.06) for deaths (8% vs 10%).
  - 0.77 (95% CI 0.66–0.91) for death or dependency (24% vs 31%).
- Grade, age, amount of blood, and lumen size had no effect on relative risks.
- Rebleeding up to 1 year was seen in 22 vs 21. A higher risk of bleeding postcoiling was offset by a greater delay before neurosurgery, during which some preprocedure rebleeds occurred.
- Long-term follow-up of 2004 patients for a mean 9 years (range 6–14 years) confirmed low rebleeding risk regardless of method used. More than 1 year after treatment there were 10 rebleeds from the treated aneurysm in the coiling group and three in the clipping group. A further 10 rebleeds occurred from untreated or new aneurysms. The risk of death at 5 years was significantly lower in the coiling group (11%) than in the clipping group (14%; RR 0.77, 95% CI 0.61–0.98). The proportion of survivors at 5 years who were independent in each group was the same: coiling group 83% vs clipping group 82%. Retreatment was required in 17% of coiled patients and 4% of clipped patients. 1-year survivors were at increased risk of death compared with the general population (RR 1.57, 95% CI 1.32–1.82).
- In technically-suitable aneurysms, treated in centres with sufficient expertise, endovascular coiling improves the chances of independent survival. Patients treated by coiling need follow-up reimaging annually (MRA or CTA).

Lancet 2002; **360**:1267–74.
Stroke 2007; **38**:1538–44.
Lancet Neurology 2009; **8**:427–33.

Non-operative management

- In perimesencephalic SAH, angiography is advised, but usually there is no aneurysm. Treat the headache and mobilize.
- In (proven or presumed) aneurysmal SAH:
  - Conservative management is reserved for patients too ill to withstand surgery (WFNS grades 3–5), with severe comorbidity, or where there are particular technical operative risks. The neurosurgeon (and anaesthetist) should be the ones to decide this.
  - Consider coiling where fitness for open surgery is in doubt.
  - Otherwise, bed rest for 3 weeks.
  - Treat headache (paracetamol, codeine), give stool softeners (sodium docusate 200mg bd).
  - General care of the unconscious or very ill patient—pressure areas, nutrition.
  - Later investigation and surgery may be possible for initially poor-grade patients who subsequently improve.
  - Mortality is very high.

Neurological complications

Neurological complications of SAH are listed in Table 4.2.

There are two types of hydrocephalus:
- Early obstructive hydrocephalus due to blood clots in the ventricular system. Occurs within 7 days of SAH. Ventriculostomy can be life saving, but increases the risk of rebleeding (reduced counter pressure).
- Later communicating hydrocephalus. May be due to blood within the basal cisterns or obstruction of the arachnoid villi. Seen in 10–20% over following weeks and months. This needs ventriculoperitoneal shunting.
- Suspect it in any patient with SAH who develops one or more of:
  - Headache.
  - Gradual deterioration of consciousness.
  - Impairment of cognitive function.
  - Incontinence.
  - Gait ataxia.

Table 4.2 Neurological complications of SAH

Complication	Features	Action
Re-bleeding	Sudden worsening of headache with or without loss of consciousness. 20% on the first day, 40% in the first month (without intervention). Ongoing risk without surgery is high. 1/3 have initial respiratory arrest, of whom half recover spontaneous respiration within 24h. 50% mortality	Repeat CT scan (shows rebleed in 80%). Exclude other causes of decreased level of consciousness (found in 1/3). Ventilation is justified for respiratory arrest. Consider emergency surgery for aneurysm clipping
Cerebral ischaemia (vasospasm)	About 25% incidence, usually between days 4–12, peaking at days 6–8, resolving over 2–4 weeks. 25% get focal deficits, 25% drowsiness, 50% both. 25% die. 10% of survivors severely disabled	Urgent 'triple H'—hypervolaemia, haemodilution, hypertension. Transfer to HDU/ITU. Arterial line, central venous pressure monitoring. Volume expand with albumin (500mL 5%). Stop nimodipine. Increase BP 20–40mmHg with inotropes. Repeat CT. Discuss with interventional neuroradiology
Hydrocephalus	20% of unoperated patients. Half are initially alert. By time of diagnosis 70–90% drowsy, more as time goes by. May have small pupils, headache, or confusion	Discuss with neurosurgeon. If alert or not too drowsy wait and see for 24h. Half improve, but may fluctuate. Consider serial LP over 10 days if no obstruction, brain shift, haematoma, or intraventricular haemorrhage on CT (remove 20mL each time, target closing pressure 15cmH$_2$O). Otherwise external drainage, at risk of increased rebleeding, and infection
Expanding haematoma	Progressive drowsiness over first few days	Consider urgent surgical evacuation. Otherwise supportive only
Epilepsy	10% within a month, mostly early	Terminate with IV lorazepam, diazepam, or phenytoin. IV phenytoin maintenance

Non-neurological complications

- Acute MI. Transient ECG changes, and histological subendocardial infarction, are very common.
- Cardiac arrhythmias, including ventricular tachycardia. Rarely needs specific treatment.
- Acute pulmonary oedema. Rapid onset, usually in severe SAH. Treat with oxygen, diuretics, or ventilation.
- Reactive hypertension.
- Delirium due to drugs, alcohol, or benzodiazepine withdrawal, or medical complications.
- Gastric ulcer (stress ulcer) with or without bleeding.
- Hyponatraemia and reduced plasma volume:
  - Develops 2nd–10th day.
  - Usually caused by natriuresis (cerebral salt wasting), rather than SIADH, although both are possible.
  - 10% have serum sodium concentration <125mmol/L.
  - Severe hyponatraemia causes drowsiness, irritability, confusion, and seizures.
  - 30% lose >10% of plasma volume. Reduced plasma volume may reduce cerebral perfusion, and contribute to delayed cerebral ischaemia.
  - Anticipate the problem by giving saline, or dextrose saline.
  - Strict fluid balance monitoring. Insert a urinary catheter if need be, and may need to monitor central venous pressure. Give albumen if crystalloid is insufficient to maintain filling pressure.
  - If using more than isotonic saline in severe hyponatraemia beware of over-rapid (>0.5mmol/L per hour) correction which can lead to central pontine myelinolysis.
  - Add fludrocortisone 100–300mcg/day if sodium does not increase.

Summary

1. Definitive SAH management is specialized, and involves neurosurgeons and neuroradiologists. Consult urgently with a neurosurgeon.
2. The initial priority is making the diagnosis. All patients with sudden-onset persisting headache need a CT head scan, and lumbar puncture (after 12h) if this is not diagnostic.
3. Oral (or nasogastric) nimodipine improves outcomes.
4. Pain control, fluid and electrolyte management, and complications need special attention. Manage in a high dependency ward. Avoid sedative drugs.
5. Watch for deterioration (rebleeding, hydrocephalus, ischaemia, fitting).
6. Patients in 'good grades' (initially alert) require angiography and work-up for clipping or coiling of the aneurysm.
7. Patients with poor prognosis or not fit for surgery may subsequently recover enough to allow intervention.

Chapter 5

Neuroimaging in stroke

Introduction

- Options for brain imaging include CT and MRI.
- In addition, intracranial haemorrhage (especially SAH, but also primary intracerebral haemorrhage), and work-up for carotid endarterectomy, require vascular imaging (duplex scanning, conventional angiography, MRA or contrast CTA).
- Suspected arterial dissection requires imaging by MRI/MRA, CTA, or conventional angiography.

This chapter concentrates on the basics of brain imaging. It does not aim to make you into a neuroradiologist. It will help you understand the role of imaging and techniques employed, as an aid to intelligent ordering and interpretation of results.

By convention, the left side of the brain anatomically appears on the right side of the scan (the image is seen as if looked at from the feet upwards, with the patient on his or her back).

Computed tomography (CT)

CT scanning of the brain is the best imaging technique for initial investigation of acute stroke.

A standard CT scan consists of axial images through the brain. It is made by moving an X-ray beam synchronously with detectors across a slice of the brain. The X-rays transmitted through an element, or pixel, of the slice (<1mm) is processed by a computer, which gives a numerical value to its density. The range of the densities are measured as Hounsfield numbers, with values of −1000, 0, and +1000 for air, water, and bone respectively. Differences in X-ray attenuation make it possible to differentiate normal and infarcted tissue, clotted or extravasated blood, tumour, or oedema.

In selected situations, IV injection of a non-ionic iodinated contrast agent is given to demonstrate breakdown of the blood–brain barrier or abnormal vessels, or to get a CTA.

Advantages and disadvantages of CT brain scanning

Advantages
- Widely available and non-invasive.
- Fast.
- Good sensitivity for many neurological conditions, including:
  - Cerebral infarction.
  - Intracranial bleeding:
    - primary and secondary intracerebral haemorrhage (Figs. 5.1–5.4).
    - subarachnoid haemorrhage (Fig. 5.5).
    - subdural haematoma (Figs. 5.6 and 5.7).
    - extradural haematoma.
  - Brain tumours (Fig. 5.8).
  - Cerebral abscess (Fig. 5.9).
  - Midline shift (Figs. 5.1, 5.6, 5.7, and 5.8; also see 📖 Fig. 2.1, p.45).
  - Hydrocephalus (Fig. 5.5).
  - Brain atrophy.
  - Cerebral trauma.

Disadvantages
- Relatively heavy radiation dose (in context, more a theoretical than practical problem).
- Early (<6–8h) infarction may not be visible.
- Does not show lesions involving brainstem or other parts of the brain within the posterior fossa very clearly.
- Insensitive to small lesions (<1cm).
- May miss some lesions such as:
  - Isodense subdural haematoma.
  - Low attenuation lesions near the skull.
  - Multiple sclerosis plaques.
  - Haemorrhage after 2 weeks.

CT scanning and intracranial haemorrhages

- Acute haemorrhage is visible on CT scan immediately. Recent blood clot (Fig. 5.10a—hyperdense MCA), bleeding within the brain parenchyma (Figs. 5.1–5.3), ventricular system (Fig. 5.4), subarachnoid space (Fig. 5.5), subdural (Fig. 5.6), or extradural spaces appear as hyperdensity, i.e. whiter than the brain parenchyma. This allows positive diagnosis of haemorrhagic stroke, and its exclusion. Acute subdural haemorrhage is seen as a hyperdense crescent, and chronic subdural haemorrhage as an area of low attenuation beneath the skull vault compressing the brain from outside (Figs. 5.6 and 5.7).
- The area of the increased density can be of any size or shape in patients with intracerebral bleeding, and often is surrounded by an area of low attenuation (darker) due to oedema, ischaemia, or clot retraction (Figs. 5.1 and 5.2).
- When the haemorrhage is large, it may cause midline shift (Fig. 5.1).
- Large supratentorial haematomas may cause herniation of:
  - The temporal lobe through the tentorial hiatus and compression of the brainstem.
  - The ipsilateral parasagittal cortex under the falx, compressing the ipsilateral lateral ventricle (e.g. Fig. 5.1) and may cause hydrocephalus of the contralateral lateral ventricle.
- Primary or secondary intracerebral bleeds may be associated with intraventricular bleeding (indicating poor prognosis) (Fig. 5.4). This can cause hydrocephalus by obstructing the CSF flow.
- Hypertensive bleeds tend to be in the basal ganglia, pons, or cerebellum (Figs. 5.2–5.4).
- Lobar bleeds tend to occur from aneurysms, AVMs, clotting disorders, or amyloid angiopathy (Fig. 5.1).
- Within few days to few weeks, the haematoma becomes isodense and subsequently hypodense (dark). Similar CT scan changes occur with other types of intracranial bleeding including subdural haematoma (Fig. 5.7).
- IV contrast may help to diagnose haemorrhages into tumours which otherwise may be missed.
- After about a week, IV contrast may show a ring enhancement around the haematoma, which can mimic cerebral tumour or abscess.

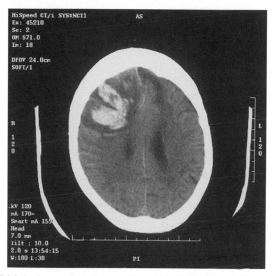

Fig. 5.1 Lobar haemorrhage due to amyloid angiopathy. Unenhanced CT head scan. Anteriorly, there is subfalcine herniation causing midline shift.

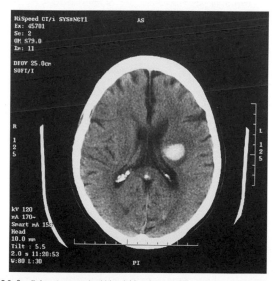

Fig. 5.2 Small deep intracerebral bleed. Unenhanced CT head. The patient presented with a dense right hemiparesis, indistinguishable clinically from a lacunar infarct.

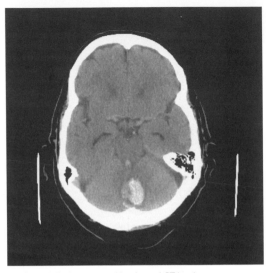

Fig. 5.3 Left cerebellar haematoma. Unenhanced CT head.

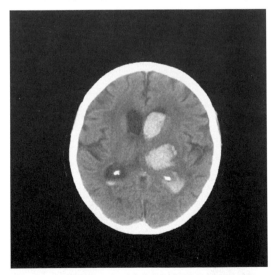

Fig. 5.4 Intracerebral bleed (based on left thalamus) with intraventricular extension. Unenhanced CT head. Blood can be seen in the posterior horn of the right lateral ventricle.

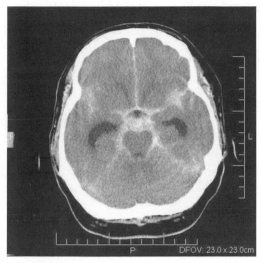

Fig. 5.5 SAH. Unenhanced CT head. Extensive blood around the base of the brain secondary to a ruptured basilar aneurysm, and acute hydrocephalus.

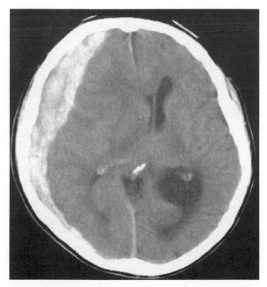

Fig. 5.6 Acute subdural haematoma. A crescent of bright (acute) blood seen on the right compressing the underlying brain, and causing midline shift.

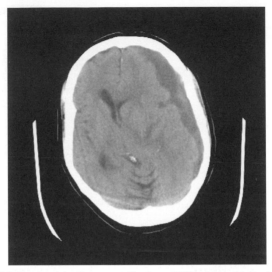

Fig. 5.7 Chronic subdural haematoma. Unenhanced CT head. Large low-density left chronic subdural haematoma, compressing the brain, and causing midline shift.

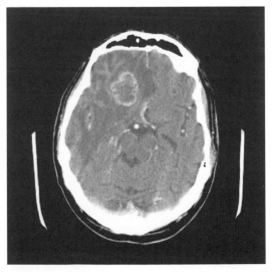

Fig. 5.8 Right frontal lobe metastasis from lung cancer. CT head scan post contrast. There is a craggy ring enhancing lesion in the right frontal lobe with surrounding oedema, causing midline shift.

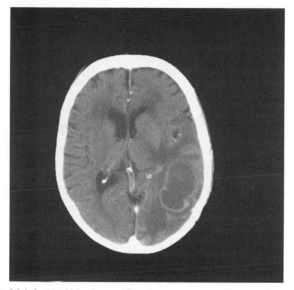

Fig. 5.9 Left parietal lobe abscess. CT head scan post contrast. There is a thin walled ring enhancing lesion with surrounding oedema.

CT scanning for cerebral infarction

- In the first 24h, the CT scan may be normal in patients with cerebral infarction, particularly those with small lesions. Up to 40% of stroke patients may never have a visible lesion on CT.
- Ischaemic changes may be seen as early as 1h after stroke onset, but are seen more reliably after 3–6h. Early signs of ischaemia include:
  - Occluded vessel—hyperdense middle cerebral (or other) artery: due to a clot in the artery (seen in 20–40%, but less reliable in elderly people) (Fig. 5.10a).
  - Loss of grey–white matter differentiation, particularly loss of visualization of the insular ribbon (Fig. 5.10b).
  - Effacement of overlying cortical sulci (mass effect due to oedema) (Fig. 5.10b).
  - Loss of outline of the lentiform nucleus of the basal ganglia (Fig. 5.10c).
  - Low density in the cortex and subcortical white matter (Fig. 5.10c).
- The Alberta Stroke Programme Early CT Score(ASPECTS) is a standardized, semiquantified, system for rating early MCA territory ischaemia, that promotes systematic reading of a scan, and provides prognostic information (Box 5.1 and Fig. 5.11).
- Established cerebral infarction is seen as an area of low attenuation which is due to increased water content of the cells (Figs. 5.12–5.15). If the infarction is extensive, the brain swelling and oedema may occur within the first 24h causing midline shift (see 📖 Fig. 5.7, p.118).
- Haemorrhagic transformation may occur and will be shown as increased density (white) at the centre of the infarction, either:
  - A frank haematoma.
  - A diffuse speckled petechial pattern.
- During the 2nd week the infarction increases in density and may become isodense, making the infarcted area similar to the surrounding brain.
- Brainstem and cerebellar infarctions may be visible (Fig. 5.14) but if they are small, can be difficult to visualize due to bone artefacts.
- Old infarctions are seen as well-demarcated hypodense lesions (holes) with similar density to that of the CSF.

(a) (b)

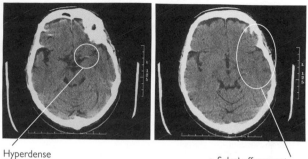

Hyperdense
MCA sign

- Sulcal effacement
- Loss of insular ribbon
- Subtle hypodensity

(c)

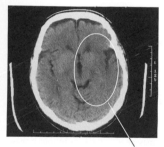

- Loss of definition of lentiform nucleus
- Loss of grey–white differentiation

Fig. 5.10 Early changes of acute infarction, left MCA territory. Unenhanced CT head. a) Hyperdense MCA sign. b) Sulcal effacement (the swollen brain presses the sulci together, including the Sylvian fissure). c) Subtle hypodensity, loss of definition of the lentiform nucleus.

Box 5.1 The Alberta Stroke Programme Early CT Score (ASPECTS)

ASPECTS is a standardized CT scoring system, quantifying damage to the MCA territory, in acute ischaemic strokes. The score divides the MCA territory into 10 regions of interest, derived from two CT slices. One slice is at the level of the thalamus and basal ganglia (deep structures plus M1 to M3), and one at the level of the ventricles immediately above the basal ganglia (M4 to M6).

The 10 regions are:
- Caudate (C).
- Lentiform nucleus (putamen) (L).
- Internal capsule (IC).
- Insular cortex (I).
- M1: anterior MCA cortex (frontal operculum).
- M2: MCA cortex lateral to insular ribbon (anterior temporal lobe).
- M3: posterior MCA cortex (posterior temporal lobe).
- M4: anterior MCA territory immediately superior to M1.
- M5: lateral MCA territory immediately superior to M2.
- M6: posterior MCA territory immediately superior to M3.

These are shown in Fig. 5.11.

1 point is subtracted from an initial score of 10, for each region in which there is evidence of infarction (focal swelling or parenchymal hypoattenuation).

In a population of stroke patients receiving thrombolysis, baseline ASPECTS score correlated strongly with baseline NIHSS score. A baseline ASPECTS of ≤7 discriminated likely independence from death or dependence at 3 months. Only 3 of 65 patients with a score of 7 or less recovered to independence (mRS 0–2), compared with 71 of 89 with a score of >7. Sensitivity for good outcome was 0.78, specificity 0.96.

ASPECTS prompts the systematic examination of a scan for abnormalities. It is simple and reliable, and has good predictive properties, but tells you little about whether thrombolysis is indicated or not.

Lancet 2000; **355**:1670–74.

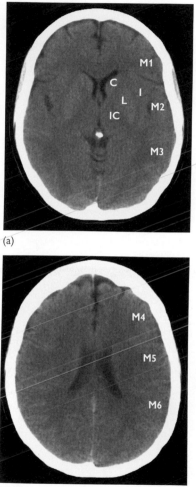

Fig. 5.11 Normal CT head showing 10 regions of interests for ASPECTS score.
a) C head of caudate, L lentiform nucleus, IC internal capsule, I insular cortex, M1 to M3 lower MCA cortex. b) M4 to M6 upper MCA cortex.

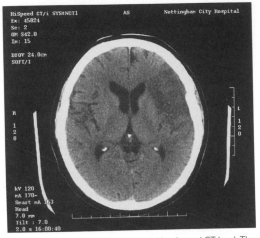

Fig. 5.12 MCA territory infarct, 24h after onset. Unenhanced CT head. There is a large low attenuation area in the left frontal region.

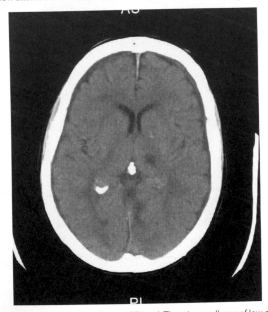

Fig. 5.13 Lacunar infarct. Unenhanced CT head. There is a small area of low density in the left thalamus.

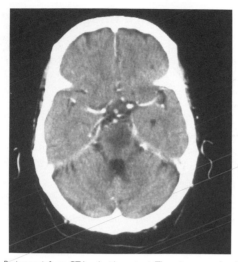

Fig. 5.14 Brainstem infarct. CT head with contrast. There is a non-enhancing low attenuation area in the left side of the pons and midbrain. The MCA and basilar artery can be clearly seen.

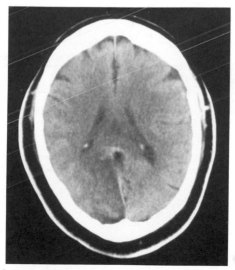

Fig. 5.15 Occipital cortex infarct. Unenhanced CT head. There is a low attenuation area in the right occipital region. The anatomical distribution is that of the right posterior cerebral artery.

Magnetic resonance imaging (MRI)

MRI detects the presence, and mobility, of hydrogen atoms. T1-weighted images show brain structure (fat is white, water and bone black). T2-weighted images show areas with high water content as white (e.g. CSF, infarction, oedema).

Advantages

- Radiation free.
- The pictures are technically superior (better spatial resolution).
- More sensitive for cerebral infarction, especially in the posterior fossa and lacunar infarction.
- Diffusion weighted images (DWI) are very sensitive to early infarction (30min after onset; Figs. 5.16 and 5.17). Absence of a DWI lesion almost excludes acute infarction.
- More sensitive for micro haemorrhages, vascular malformations, and tumour underlying a bleed. Microbleeding may indicate angiopathy with increased risk of haemorrhagic transformation after antithrombotic and thrombolytic therapy, but the practical importance of this in decision making is still unclear.
- MRA can be performed at the same time (without the need for contrast, although using contrast gives better sensitivity) (see Fig 1.3a,b, p.27).
- Can detect sites of old haemorrhage (through persisting haemoglobin breakdown products).
- Can detect vasculitis.

Disadvantages

- Relatively slow and noisy, with poorer access for monitoring. 10% of patients cannot be examined due to claustrophobia. A further 10% have another contraindication (agitation, cardiorespiratory instability, vomiting, metallic implants). Scan times are getting much quicker, however.
- As sensitive as CT in detecting intracerebral haemorrhage, but can be more difficult to interpret for non-neuroradiologists.
- Cranial MRI scanning may be contraindicated in patients with metallic foreign bodies, e.g. stents and heart valves, intracranial metal aneurysm clips, pacemakers, cochlear implants, and programmable hydrocephalus shunts. All possible metallic foreign bodies and prostheses (including intraocular metallic foreign bodies) should be notified in advance to the scanning department for advice regarding compatibility.

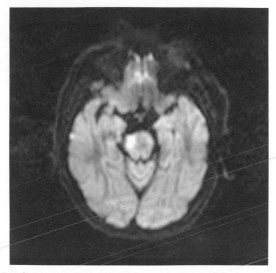

Fig. 5.16 Right pontine infarct. MRI diffusion-weighted image. The infarct shows as a bright spot in the brainstem.

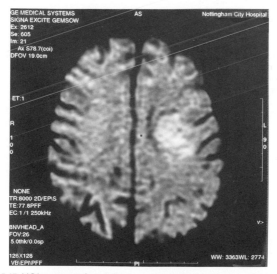

Fig. 5.17 MCA territory infarct. Diffusion-weighted MRI showing acute infarction in the left frontal lobe.

Infarction on MRI

- DWI is very sensitive for acute infarction. 50% of TIAs lasting >30min, and most TIAs and strokes lasting >1h show as a distinctive bright lesion on DWI (see 📖 Figs. 5.16 and 5.17, p.127). This is especially useful for lacunar and brainstem strokes, recurrent strokes and strokes occurring where there is extensive subcortical white matter ischaemic change (leukoaraiosis).
- Other early signs are a loss of the normal flow void in the affected artery (immediate), swelling on T1, and intense bright signal on T2 (6h), which remains bright for 1–2 weeks (Figs. 5.18 and 5.19; also see 📖 Fig. 1.3d, p.27).
- After this lesions may become isointense with normal brain.
- After several weeks infarcts look like CSF (dark T1, bright T2).

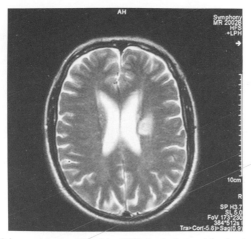

Fig. 5.18 Lacunar infarction. T2-weighted MRI showing lacunar infarction deep in the corona radiata (white matter projection of the internal capsule).

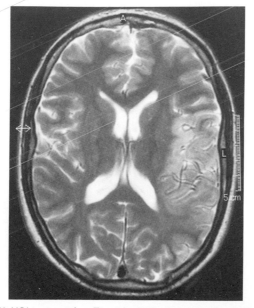

5.19 MCA territory infarct. T2-weighted MRI, a large left frontoparietal infarct.

Haemorrhage on MRI

- MRI signals vary according to the age of the haemorrhage, but this should not be a problem in experienced hands, and with special MR sequences (T2* or gradient echo).
- Early appearances (hyperacute) may be confused with infarction. There may be a bright core on T2 images, with a dark rim of deoxyhaemoglobin.
- After about 24h the blood shows as dark on both T1 and T2 images due to deoxyhaemoglobin formation (acute phase; Figs. 5.20 and 5.21).
- Over the next few days the T1 image becomes bright again as methaemoglobin forms (early subacute; Figs. 5.22 and 5.23). The lesion remains dark on T2.
- After a week both T1 and T2 images are bright (late subacute; Figs. 5.24 and 5.25).
- After several weeks a dark ring (haemosiderin) forms around the haemorrhage on T1. This is seen even more intensely on T2 images, and persists (useful in diagnosing a late presentation; Figs. 5.26 and 5.27).
- T2* images are very sensitive to showing blood breakdown products (Fig. 5.28), and can show microbleeds that are not visible on T1 or T2 images (Fig. 5.29).

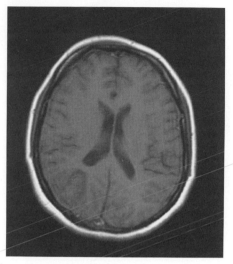

Fig. 5.20 Acute right parietal lobe bleed, 3 days after onset. The haematoma is hypointense (dark) on T1-weighted images. (Image courtesy of Dr Sami Khan).

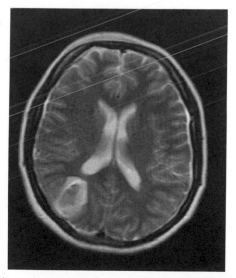

Fig. 5.21 Acute right parietal lobe bleed, 3 days after onset. The haematoma is coming hypointense (dark) on the T2-weighted image as well. (Image courtesy of Sami Khan).

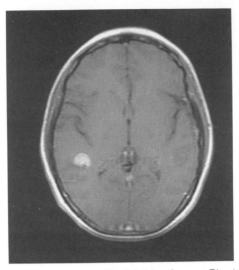

Fig. 5.22 Early subacute right parietal bleed, 3–7 days after onset. T1-weighted image. The haematoma is hyperintense (bright) due to methaemoglobin formation. (Image courtesy of Dr Sami Khan).

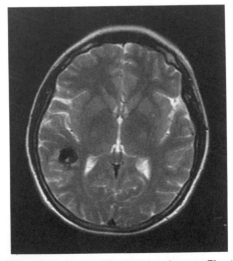

Fig. 5.23 Early subacute right parietal bleed, 3–7 days after onset. T2-weighted image. The haematoma is hypointense (dark). (Image courtesy of Dr Sami Khan).

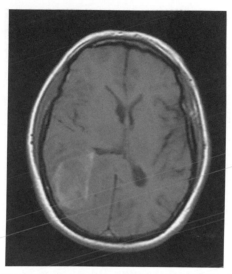

Fig. 5.24 Late subacute right parietal bleed, 7–14 days after onset. T1-weighted image. The haematoma is hyperintense (bright). (Image courtesy of Dr Sami Khan).

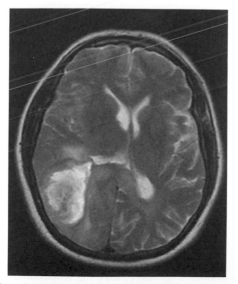

Fig. 5.25 Late subacute right parietal bleed, 7–14 days after onset. T2-weighted image. The haematoma is now hyperintense (bright). (Image courtesy of Dr Sami Khan).

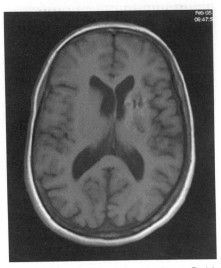

Fig. 5.26 Chronic left basal ganglion bleed. T1-weighted image. Dark haemosiderin is seen. (Image courtesy of Dr Sami Khan).

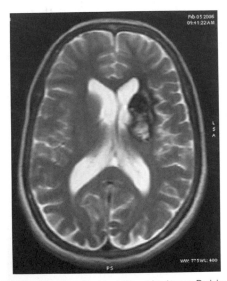

Fig. 5.27 Chronic left basal ganglion bleed. T2-weighted image. Dark haemosiderin is seen. (Image courtesy of Dr Sami Khan).

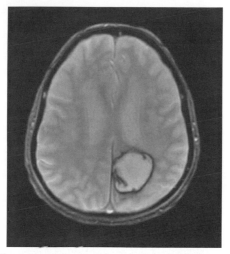

Fig. 5.28 Chronic bleed, left parietal lobe, 10 weeks after onset. T2* image. The haematoma cavity is bright with an intensely dark haemosiderin rim.

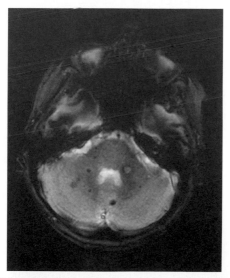

Fig. 5.29 Multiple cavernomas in the cerebellum showing evidence of microbleeding (black dots). The T1- and T2-weighted images looked normal. (Image courtesy of Dr Sami Khan).

Vascular imaging

- Conventional catheter angiography is the gold standard and has high sensitivity for detecting arterial stenosis, intracranial vascular aneurysms and malformations, and tumours. It is most useful prior to and following radiological intervention (coiling, stenting, embolizing, intra-arterial thrombolysis, or mechanical clot retrieval), for which vascular access is required anyway. It is also used when doubt remains that impacts on clinical decision-making following less invasive imaging. However, the procedure is invasive, and carries a procedure-related mortality and stroke risk (0.1% for diagnostic angiography alone).
- Carotid duplex scanning uses ultrasound to examine the structure of the artery wall, including intima–media thickness, atheromatous plaque and ulceration, and Doppler to determine flow velocity. From this, degree of stenosis is estimated. Initially intended as a rapidly available screening test, to be followed up with angiography, some surgeons will perform carotid endarterctomy on the basis of duplex findings alone. However, sensitivity and specificity for operable stenosis are both 0.8–0.9—some false positives and negatives occur. The technique requires careful training and audit. Different operators do not always agree on degree of stenosis, and some are better at it than others.
- CTA requires injection of non-iodinated contrast. The technique is rapid, has good resolution, and can be used to identify carotid or vertebral stenosis, intracranial aneurysms, and vascular malformations. A related technique, CT perfusion scanning, can delineate areas of loss of blood flow (sometimes useful in thrombolysis decisions; Fig. 5.30). CT venography can be used to diagnose venous sinus thrombosis. Contrast-induced nephropathy is a risk in those with poor renal function—always tell the imaging department about renal function on requests.
- MRA is also a convenient add-on to other MRI, with similar indications to CTA. Some images ('time of flight') can be reconstructed without the use of contrast, but IV gadolinium contrast increases definition and sensitivity (see 📖 Fig. 1.3a,b, p.27). Magnetic resonance venography can be performed to detect venous sinus thrombosis. Some contrast agents have been associated with systemic fibrosis in patients with poor renal function—always tell the imaging department about renal function on requests.
- MR diffusion–perfusion mismatch (a difference in area of underperfusion on perfusion scan, and acute infarction on DWI) is hypothesized to represent potentially salvageable 'ischaemic penumbra', that may be amenable to reperfusion by thrombolysis. Trials attempting to exploit this (to extend the time window for thrombolysis and spare patients with no mismatch from futile treatment) have been inconclusive.
- Transcranial Doppler uses bone windows, most importantly across the temporal bone, to examine blood flow in intracranial arteries. Patterns of blood flow can suggest occlusion, or intracranial stenosis, and examine collateral flow around the circle of Willis. One application is to establish rapidly whether reperfusion has occurred (or not) after thrombolysis. The technique is not widely used in the UK.

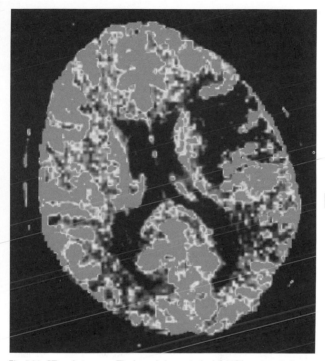

Fig. 5.30 CT perfusion scan. The large dark area in the left MCA territory indicates lack of perfusion due to acute MCA occlusion.

Summary

1. CT head scan is the initial investigation of choice. It should be performed urgently if bleeding, SAH, tumour, or abscess is suspected, if there is unexplained coma, or thrombolysis is being considered. Otherwise, it should be performed within 24h of onset. It can distinguish infarcts from bleeds, and identify most non-vascular pathologies mimicking stroke.

2. CT scan may not detect early infarction, but is very sensitive for detecting bleeds.

3. MRI is especially useful in examining the posterior fossa, and is more sensitive than CT in identifying lacunar infarcts. Diffusion-weighted images have excellent sensitivity very early after infarction.

4. Vascular imaging uses duplex ultrasound as the main screening modality for the carotid arteries. CTA or MRA are confirmatory tests for carotid disease, or for imaging the vertebrobasilar system, and intracranial vessels.

5. Discuss urgent, contentious, difficult, or unusual requests with the radiologist.

Making difficult decisions

Consent

Most healthcare interventions require consent. Merely touching someone without their permission may constitute 'battery'. Doing anything which might (to the legal mind) constitute an injury, may be an assault. Health professionals are unused to thinking like this, but some patients, lawyers, and governments do.

The key points are:
- You must get consent before you examine, investigate, treat, or otherwise care for a competent adult patient.
- Consent may be *explicit* (permission asked and granted), or *implied* (the patient comes to you voluntarily, asks for help, cooperates, and does not object to what you are proposing or doing, e.g. holding his or her arm out so you can take blood).
- Explicit consent can be *written*, or *verbal*, and both are equally valid (although the latter is harder to prove).
- An adult is anyone over the age of 18 years. In the UK, between ages 16 and 18, and for younger children who can understand what is involved (so-called 'Gillick-competent' minors), matters are more complicated. The patient can give his or her own consent, as can a parent, but he or she cannot withhold consent (for arcane legal reasons). Otherwise, a parent must consent, except in an emergency.
- Always assume an adult is competent (or '*has capacity*') to give or withhold consent unless you can demonstrate otherwise.
- Patients may be competent to make some decisions, but not others, and their ability to consent may vary with time. Patients may change their mind about consenting (or not consenting).
- A decision which you find surprising, or with which you disagree, does not prove that the patient does not have capacity. Competent adults may refuse any treatment, even if it would clearly benefit their health, unless it is treatment of a mental illness and they are detained under the Mental Health Act.
- Consent must be 'informed'—otherwise it is invalid. This means patients need sufficient information to be able to come to a decision, such as benefits and risks, and possible alternative treatments.
- Consent must also be voluntary—not under any duress from relatives, friends, or staff.
- A representative may have been legally appointed who has authority to take decisions for an incapacitated patient (in England, the holder of a health and welfare Lasting Power of Attorney). Otherwise, no one can give consent on behalf of an adult who does not have capacity to consent. They may be treated if it is in their 'best interests'.

Capacity

Assessing capacity is asking whether someone can understand and use information necessary to make a decision. To have capacity to consent a patient must:

- Understand the nature, purpose, and effects of the treatment.
- Understand any adverse effects, any alternative treatments, and the consequences of refusal.
- Be able to take in, retain, believe, and weigh up the information to make a judgement.
- Communicate a decision.
- Do so free from undue pressure.

Understanding need only be in broad terms. This is fortunate, as you might imagine that on these criteria a large proportion of your patients cannot give their own consent. Patients may be able to consent to some things, but not others.

How to make decisions

Four factors are considered in the widely-accepted ethical framework called 'principlism':
- Beneficence, or doing good ('benefits')
- Non-maleficence, or avoiding harm ('burdens or risks')
- Autonomy
- Justice, or equity.

The first two define whether an intervention is *effective* or not—is it technically feasible? Unless the likely good from a procedure outweighs the likely harm, or at least justifies it, it is not effective. Good and harm is judged in terms of effect on length of life, curing diseases, reducing symptoms or increasing abilities, avoiding complications and side-effects, and the short-term unpleasantness or debility associated with the procedure.

If a procedure is ineffective, or is highly unlikely to have its desired effect, it is said to be *futile*. In these cases consent is not generally an issue, as futile interventions should not be offered to patients. There may still be a need for, or an obligation to give, an explanation of why potential treatments are not being offered.

Assuming that there is a reasonable prospect of an intervention doing more good than harm, next consider *autonomy*. This is essentially the same as asking consent.

How you proceed depends on whether the patient has capacity to decide or not. Autonomy does not dictate that a futile procedure should be undertaken, even if the patient wants it, but otherwise the autonomy of competent patients must be respected. They can exercise it by refusing a treatment that might be effective. The only way of finding out what a patient wants is to ask them.

If a patient can give you the information you need, do not ask relatives or friends first. It is technically a breach of *confidentiality* to discuss things without the patient's permission, and their opinions may not accurately reflect those of the patient. If a patient does not have capacity, then we can still respect autonomy by trying to find out what they would have wanted (see 📖 p.144).

Equity and justice refer to two things:
- *Non-discrimination*; on the basis of things that should have no influence on decision making (sex, race, religion, political views, disability, age).
- *Rationing*, or fair shares; available resources must be used to maximize the good done overall to the greatest number of people. This is really the responsibility of politicians and health administrators. It can make life difficult for doctors, because the clinical ethic demands that we do our best for the patient in front of us, ideally without taking account of resource issues. As a general rule use common sense.

Best interest

The idea of 'best interest' applies where a patient does not have capacity to give or withhold consent (Box 6.1). In the UK, a treatment may be legally given, despite lack of consent, if it is in the patient's best interest, so long as there is no formal advance decision to refuse treatment, no holder of a health and welfare Lasting Power of Attorney, nor court appointed deputy (any of which must be consulted and the views expressed respected).

Assessment of best interest in UK law actually represents quite a libertarian position. The right of a vulnerable person to make unwise decisions is prioritized above that of protection from risk of harm or exploitation, although the Act appears to presuppose that the proposed course of action is both practicable and reasonably safe. In general, the courts are supportive of professionals acting sensibly and in good faith.

The technical issue of effectiveness still holds—the benefits of treatment must justify the burdens. One published formulation, which is useful when discussing the issues with involved parties (staff, relatives), is:

- Is the proposed treatment likely to lead to a length and quality of life that the patient would have found acceptable?

This introduces ideas beyond the likely clinical outcome (length and quality of life). They include a need to respect the wishes of the patient. There are several levels of information:

- An *advanced directive*, *advanced decision to refuse treatment*, or *living will*, may legally define in some detail what the patient would or would not have wanted done (✆ http://www.adrtnhs.co.uk/). This has the force of law. Unfortunately very few people have made these (have you?). There may be some doubt as to whether the exact circumstances intended by the patient actually apply.
- A *proxy judgement*: someone may be able to tell you what the patient would have said, because they had discussed the issues previously. The degree of uncertainty mounts when the exact circumstances have not been discussed, but opinions may still be known in general terms. This often comes down to asking 'knowing the person as you do, what do you think they would have wanted?'—which is a pretty rough and ready assessment of opinion.
- A *substitute judgement*: this asks what the informant (relative, friend, or staff member) would want in this situation. This may be useful when someone is of a particular religious faith, where general principles are well known. Staff making this judgement are essentially saying 'as a fellow human being what would I have wanted?' This has some validity, but opinions do vary widely.

Be careful, as research has shown that some people with a condition view it as less bad than do staff members, relatives, or members of the general population (who are the most averse to descriptions of severe disability). The majority of the population, however, when asked, rate living with a severe stroke as bad as death, or worse than death. A minority disagree.

Avoid giving the impression that you are asking family members to make life or death decisions. Concentrate on asking what the patient would have wanted were they able to given their opinion. There is a legal duty to consult, and take views into account, but relatives' views are not binding (if you have a very good reason for deciding otherwise). Moreover, it is unfair to burden families with further distress and possible guilt, when they are having to cope with severe illness in a close relative.

Decision making requires some knowledge about:
• The condition.
• Its natural history.
• The effectiveness of treatment.
• What the patient would have wanted you to do.

There is usually uncertainty about all of these, which makes life difficult, and good judgement important. When the ethical framework is properly applied it is quite simple, and many nurses and junior doctors will have the necessary knowledge and skills. However, these discussions should usually involve the most senior doctor available. You should always be able to expect support, both in making decisions and discussing them, or their consequences, if you need it.

Ultimate responsibility for deciding on best interest, and formally declaring it to be so, rests with the consultant in charge of the case. Senior staff may want support by discussing cases with colleagues, or asking second opinions.

Box 6.1 Criteria for determining best interests in England and Wales

• Encourage participation in the decision and care.
• Respect the patient's past and present views if possible.
• Seek the opinion of family members, or others, whom it is appropriate and practical to consult.
• Use the least restrictive alternative option.
• There is a general authority to *act reasonably* on behalf of someone without capacity.

Mental Capacity Act 2005.

Advance care planning

This is intended as a means to promote and extend patient autonomy, for someone who has mental capacity, in advance of a time when it may be lost. It may take the form of an advance statement of wishes or preferences, an advance decision to refuse treatment, or the appointment of a welfare Lasting Power of Attorney. The majority of people will not want to document anything formally following discussion, although they may find the discussion process itself valuable.

The context should generally be a long-standing, trusting professional relationship. The time after a stroke will not usually be a good one for advance care planning:
- Health and function may be changing rapidly.
- Psychological consequences of stroke, including depression and cognitive impairment, may compromise judgement.
- The process of psychological adjustment may lead to dramatic changes in attitudes and values.
- The professional relationship will often be too short, and potentially open to conflicts of interest.

Some people may, however, choose the time after a stroke to consider how they would like to plan for future healthcare. The patient's GP or care home manager should be invited to contribute. Plans are usually most useful for someone who is very disabled, and would prefer to avoid readmission to hospital in the case of a deterioration. Unfortunately, many people in this situation lack mental capacity to engage in the process. The Royal College of Physicians has published sensible guidelines (http://www.rcplondon.ac.uk/pubs/epubs.aspx).

Managing decision making

We must make decisions well, be seen to make them well, and 'carry' staff and families with the process. The ideal is to reach consensus and agreement. This is often possible, by explaining the process behind decision making, and showing that the health professional is not arbitrarily 'playing God'.

Sometimes, strong convictions and emotions raise barriers to what rational thought dictates. We must be sensitive to these—acknowledge them, show you understand them, take them into account or accept them. Remember, however, that acting against the 'best interest' of someone who cannot speak for themselves is illegal. Common sense must prevail. Defining best interest is not always obvious or precise. A 'cosmetic' drip may help a relative come to terms with the impending death of a family member. Avoid being dogmatic, but you must always be ready and able to justify what you have done after the event.

Sometimes, uncertainty in decision making means we must prevaricate. A holding operation for a few days (or weeks), such as IV hydration, whilst we see which way things are turning out, is perfectly acceptable if a decision can be postponed. We are gathering more information on which to base a final judgement.

Applying this to stroke care

Capacity to consent

The main problems are:
- Coma.
- Aphasia.
- Cognitive impairment due to stroke.
- Comorbid dementia, learning disabilities, or delirium.
- Other communication problems such as deafness.
- Language barriers in non-English speakers—although the decisions are sufficiently important to justify getting a translator if no family member is bilingual and willing to help (in England this is a legal requirement under the Mental Capacity Act).

Medical interventions without consent in conditions which may only be temporary, should be limited to those required to preserve life and immediate health. In practice, this rarely applies in stroke:
- We may not know how reversible the condition will be, e.g. cognitive impairment or aphasia.
- Or how quickly it might reverse.
- Sometimes, if you are going to treat something at all, you need to treat quickly—such as antibiotics or rehydration.

As a general rule, if someone has presented to hospital, it is reasonable to give nursing and medical care (i.e. anything short of operative procedures), as you think is best practice and in their best interests, unless or until someone objects. At that point you can reassess more formally:
- Formally consider someone's capacity to consent.
- The nature of the objection.
- The likely alternatives.
- The status of the person objecting—clearly the views of the patient, a spouse, or (adult) child have more weight than those of the next-door neighbour.
- Whether someone else has relevant information or views which must be sought prior to making a decision.
- What best interest comprises.

Any proposed operative procedure (such as placing a feeding tube) should trigger the same process.

Speech and language therapists may help with decision making for patients with aphasia by assessing level of comprehension, or explaining procedures (such as PEG insertion) in the optimal way, including use of picture cards ('supported conversation').

Disturbed behaviour

The commonest scenario for apparent 'objection' to treatment is a patient who is confused—by which we mean delirious, demented, or psychotic. This may manifest itself as agitation, aggression, shouting, wandering, and interference with medical devices such as drips, feeding tubes, or urinary catheters. There may be interference with other patients.

- Make a diagnosis—from the mental state examination (alertness, evidence of hallucinations or delusions, speech, cognition) and a third-party premorbid history.
- Identify any underlying medical conditions—infections (temperature, white cell count, C-reactive protein, focal signs such as sputum or abnormal urinalysis), drugs, drug withdrawal, hypoxia, heart failure.
- Identify aggravating factors—pain, constipation, urinary retention, illusions or misinterpretations (cot sides or prison bars?), fear.
- Nurse in a light, quiet environment, away from other patients if possible. Avoid confrontation or threats (they never work), maximize sensory awareness if possible (sit out, glasses, hearing aid) and attempt diversion if behaviour is troublesome.
- Avoid sedative drugs if possible. These are effective at relieving anxiety and psychotic symptoms. If these are driving disturbed behaviour then use drugs. If we are dealing with disorientation and bewilderment in someone with dementia, then short of sedating someone to the point of immobility ('chemical strait jacket') they are unlikely to help. As a last resort be guided by the drugs in Table 6.1.
- Best interest in these circumstances is represented by those treatments necessary to maintain the safety of the patient, other patients and staff, and to address the underlying medical condition.
- In the UK psychiatrists are reluctant to use the Mental Health Act in these circumstances, but may do so, and they may need to be consulted about diagnosis and management. In the UK Deprivation of Liberty Safeguards may apply for someone with a mental disorder, who lacks capacity to decide to stay in hospital (or a care home) and whose liberty is being deprived (or is at risk of being deprived). Deprivation (as opposed to restriction) of liberty is not well defined, but consider the possibility if you or the multiprofessional team prevent someone who is asking or trying to leave.

Table 6.1 Drugs for emergency control of severely disturbed behaviour

Patient group	Try first	Try second	Max. dose in first 6h
Already on depot/ regular high-dose antipsychotics	Lorazepam 2mg IM	Repeat lorazepam, then try haloperidol 5mg IM	Lorazepam 4mg + haloperidol 18mg
Acute alcoholic withdrawal	Lorazepam 2mg IM	Repeat	Lorazepam 8mg
Frail elderly or severe respiratory disease	Haloperidol 2.5mg IM	Lorazepam 1mg IM	Lorazepam 4mg + haloperidol 10mg
Highly aroused, physically robust, adult	Lorazepam 2mg IM + haloperidol 5mg IM	Repeat	Lorazepam 4mg + haloperidol 18mg

Cardiopulmonary resuscitation (CPR)

The usual principles should apply—except that CPR and do not attempt resuscitation (DNAR) orders have got caught up with rather ill-informed press and political opinion.

The main issue is futility. Success rates to discharge after CPR attempts on coronary care units are about 50%. On general medical wards, they are perhaps 5%. Resuscitation is successful when cardiac arrest is due to ventricular tachyarrhythmias or ventricular fibrillation, which most often occurs shortly after MI.

A long list of other conditions is associated with poor (or negligible) chances of success. These include:

- Severe stroke.
- Systemic sepsis.
- Severe metabolic derangements.
- Renal failure.
- Disseminated malignancy.
- Severe anaemia.
- Severe lung disease.
- Pulmonary embolism.
- 'Severe general frailty'.

In these cases death is not due to an acute arrhythmia, and CPR is futile. For example, in severe stroke death is due to brain damage, or oedema, raised intracranial pressure and tentorial herniation, pulmonary embolism, or sepsis.

People with cerebral vascular disease often have coronary artery disease as well. If primary neurological death is not expected, and there are no overwhelming comorbidities or complications, there is no reason to expect that people with mild or moderate stroke might not benefit from CPR if they collapse unexpectedly with cardiac arrest. In these cases we adopt the 'presumption of active treatment' unless we have information to the contrary.

The patient may have told you that they would not have wanted a CPR attempt. They are quite at liberty to do so under the general rules of consent. In some cases you may like to ask. We feel that it is unduly worrying to approach all patients about their wishes routinely, although a general information sheet might be used. The issues are often not well understood, and patients may feel they are being told they are going to die, or may fear they are not valued, or might be denied other treatments. Some people are more open to these discussions than others, and things are changing rapidly as the issues are aired in the press and on television.

For patients who are not able to give their own opinions, we can ask family or close friends what the patient would have wanted were they able to say. This information can often be appended to discussions about other things. If CPR is likely futile it may be more a matter of telling than asking. Avoid the trap of asking the family what they want. It is the patient's best interest that concerns you. This is informed by what the family says, but is not determined by them. Some people value life almost at all costs (e.g. some orthodox Jews and Muslims).

Dementia, in particular, is a distressing condition, and you should think very carefully about resuscitation attempts on anyone with moderate dementia or worse.

Current UK guidelines (2007), set out in: *Decisions relating to cardiopulmonary resuscitation: A joint statement from the British Medical Association, the Resuscitation Council (UK) and the Royal College of Nursing* (℘ http://www.resus.org.uk/pages/dnar.pdf) are sensible and measured. Advice includes:

- Where death is expected and no DNAR decision has been made, healthcare professionals can decide against resuscitating at the time.
- If the clinical team believes that CPR will not restart the heart and maintain breathing, it should not be offered or attempted.
- When a clinical decision is made that CPR should not be attempted, because it will not be successful, and the patient has not expressed a wish to discuss CPR, it is neither necessary nor appropriate to initiate discussion with the patient about CPR
- Patients on whom a DNAR decision has been made, may have emergency treatment that may amount to resuscitation if a readily reversible cause is evident (such as choking).
- If a patient with capacity is at foreseeable risk of cardiac or respiratory arrest, and the healthcare team has doubts about whether the benefits of CPR would outweigh the burdens, or whether the level of recovery expected would be acceptable to the patient, this should be discussed with the patient.
- If a patient lacks capacity, previously expressed wishes should be considered when making a CPR decision. Otherwise the risks and burdens for the particular patient should be discussed with family or others close to or representing the patient.

Drips and feeding tubes

The balance sheet of potential good and potential harm is given in Table 6.2. In each case, the pros and cons will be differently balanced. Some will vary with individual opinions. This emphasizes the importance of trying to respect autonomy.

The main problem in deciding about the desirability of inserting a gastrostomy tube is *uncertainty*, about:

- Outcomes. Patients admitted with swallowing problems, which do not recover within a couple of weeks usually have had severe strokes. We know that for patients with total anterior circulation strokes, 60% will be dead within a year. 4% will recover to independence (actually fewer, if we exclude patients with initially severe deficits which recover quickly).
- How people feel about the value or worth of the likely outcomes. Most people (but not all) consider life with a severe stroke to be at least as bad as death. We are relatively poor at predicting which people will do well (on the basis of clinical features or scores based on multivariate prediction models).

- The quality of the evidence on which we have to base decisions. If someone has written an advanced decision to refuse treatment (living will) that precisely described the circumstances that pertain, there is little difficulty. Most have not. We are usually dependent on what family or friends say the person would have said were they able to say—based on what they said before, or what they think they would have said before.

Table 6.2 Benefits and burdens balance sheet for feeding decisions

Potential good	Potential harm
Relieve thirst and hunger	Risk of death or complications during insertion of PEG
Prolong life	Prolong the process of dying
Ensure best chance of making a recovery	Survival in a distressing, highly dependent state
Minimize muscle catabolism, preserving muscle mass	
Ease of nursing	

An alternative way of looking at the problem from the standpoint of 'best interest' and autonomy is to consider what the individual would give up to achieve what they want as a final outcome:
- If we want to give people their best chance of a good recovery, we should feed as many people as possible, in order not to miss those who do well despite initially poor signs.
- If the individual had expressed strong feelings about not surviving in a dependent state, they might be willing to trade the small chance of a good recovery for the avoidance of the much larger probability of surviving but being dependent.

If the patient is in a position to give an opinion, it can be discussed with them (albeit a very difficult discussion). In the end we are usually left with trying to make the best of incomplete and uncertain information. We could try to quantify the options more using formal decision analysis—but this is pretty rough and ready, and rarely done (see Ebrahim S and Harwood RH, *Stroke: Epidemiology, Evidence and Clinical Practice*, 2nd edn., Oxford University Press, 1999, p.103).

Strictly, the arguments for and against gastrostomy feeding hold for nasogastric feeding, and IV or SC fluids (except that these options have forced time-limited reviews, since cannulae must be resited and tubes replaced from time to time).

Experience shows that most patients, in whom feeding tubes are inserted after difficulties deciding, die within a few weeks. This suggests we tend to err on the side of intervention. The FOOD trials demonstrated that in practice decisions about type and timing of tube feeding have relatively little effects on outcome (see 📖 Box 3.1, p.70).

Tube feeding is legally a 'medical treatment'. Ordinary feeding by mouth is not. If we are not feeding someone, or intending to do so, it is illegal to deny them free access to food and drink, even if their swallow is 'unsafe'. Clearly if any attempt at swallowing leads to distressing aspiration, it cannot be considered in anyone's interest. Most likely the patient would not want to try after one bad experience. However, if able to say, that should be up to the patient. Sips of water are unlikely to cause undue problems. In any case, mouth care is especially important for any patient who is not swallowing.

BMA guidelines suggest that decisions to withhold or withdraw feeding or hydration should be subject to a second consultant opinion. This would be desirable in an ideal world.

Antibiotics for intercurrent infections

If someone is inevitably about to die, antibiotics serve no purpose, unless they are intended to relieve distressing symptoms. They will not usually form part of good terminal care.

The same principles of benefit, burden, and autonomy should underlie decisions to commence antibiotic treatment (implicitly at least—the framework should be held in mind even if the process is not explicit).

Antibiotic treatment for pneumonia is perhaps best thought of in probability terms rather than the more usual black and white. It is not a matter of 'active treatment—survival' vs 'no active treatment—death'. Rather, '20% chance of survival without treatment' vs '60% chance of survival with treatment'.

This is important because one unfortunate consequence of opting not to treat intercurrent infections on the grounds that the patient is terminally ill, is that the patient survives, but is further (unnecessarily) debilitated.

It should also be remembered that antibiotics have a downside as well, especially in wards where *Clostridium difficile* is endemic. Colitis associated with this produces a debilitating, long-lasting, and difficult-to-treat diarrhoea that severely undermines quality of life and rehabilitation prospects.

Who should talk to whom?

If a patient is able to do so, information and explanations should be directed at him or her. Decisions should be made by the person to whom they apply. Who else they want told, or to help or support them in making decisions (even a spouse or children), is up to them. You should not get yourself in the position of telling relatives something that you have not told a patient who is in a position to be told.

An extreme view of confidentiality does not represent good practice either, however. Strictly, we should say nothing to anyone about a patient's health state except to the person themselves, without their permission to do so. Confidentiality has to be traded-off against pragmatism and courtesy.

If a patient is severely ill, unable to communicate, or otherwise speak for themselves, naturally close relatives will be concerned and want to know what is going on. Family members may be the only source of important information about someone's medical past, and their likely wishes.

If no family is available, do not forget other sources of useful information: GPs, district nurses, neighbours, wardens (of sheltered accommodation), and social services. Watch out for visitors.

Taking the lead on decision making has traditionally fallen to doctors, but there is no especial reason why this should be so. Sometimes a problem can be introduced by one professional and followed up by another, if a difficult decision needs to be broken gently, if time is needed to think the problem through, or consult others. Senior medical staff should be available and willing to support others in this role.

Summary

1. Consent must be gained for any examination, investigation, or treatment. It may be implicit or explicit, written or verbal. For consent to be valid, sufficient information must be given for a decision to be made.

2. Assume that someone is capable of giving consent unless you can show otherwise.

3. Capacity to consent requires that the person understands the proposed treatment, can retain and weigh up the information to come to a decision, and can communicate it.

4. If someone does not have capacity, act in their best interest. But first make sure you know what that best interest is, by asking people who might be able to give the information you need.

5. If a decision is to be made, first consider feasibility—do the potential benefits outweigh the potential burdens? Then consider desirability— what does the patient want you to do, or what would the patient have wanted you to do?

6. Following a stroke, patients may not have capacity to consent, or be able to tell you what they want because of drowsiness or coma, confusion, or communication problems.

7. Many severely affected patients will die. Best interest is not necessarily served by aggressive intervention. But it might be. The trick is to determine which, and this can be hard.

Chapter 7

Terminal care

Diagnosing dying

Can we predict death?

Knowing that someone is going to die is useful, even if nothing can be done to avert it:

- Families forewarned can gather and are prepared for the worst.
- Healthcare staff can avoid futile and meddlesome treatments.
- We can concentrate on symptom relief and promoting dignity. Dignity is the right to respect, privacy, autonomy, self-worth, and ethical treatment.
- It may be possible to arrange a discharge home for terminal care if that is what everyone wants.
- Families may be more upset about a death which was not expected and about which they had no warning, than being told that death is likely in someone who subsequently recovers. There is a subtle balance between not extinguishing hope and not raising expectations. A useful aphorism is to 'hope for the best, but prepare for the worst'.

We are fairly good at recognizing that someone is about to die when they have disseminated cancer, multiple organ failure, or the later stages of neurodegenerative diseases. For other conditions it is more difficult, including stroke, and heart or respiratory failure.

All other things being equal, prolonging life is a good thing. However, we can sometimes misjudge what is for the best:

- We may be overoptimistic and intervene too vigorously when death is inevitable.
- We can fall foul of a self-fulfilling prophesy—not treating someone because we think they are dying, and they die for lack of a treatment which would otherwise have saved them.
- Sometimes palliative and potentially 'curative' approaches must proceed together. We may still want to attempt life-prolonging treatment when the chances of success are small, but not completely hopeless. However, we may have to treat many people unsuccessfully to save one life, which may not be justified if the treatment is unpleasant, uncomfortable, or compromises dignity.

Can we predict death after stroke?

No single feature, or prognostic score, determined soon after stroke onset, is sufficiently accurate to allow us to predict death (or survival) with certainty in an individual patient.

A number of clinical features are associated with a poor outcome (Box 7.1). However, there is a difference between saying that a feature, such as unconsciousness, is a poor prognostic sign, and saying that everyone with that feature does badly. For example, the 1-month mortality from primary intracerebral haemorrhage is 50%, worse than the average for stroke. But we can't conclude that everyone with a bleed dies.

The best way of describing the ability of a piece of information (feature, test result, or score) to predict an outcome is to calculate:

- The sensitivity (in this case, the proportion of people who die who have the bad feature).

- The specificity (the proportion of people who survive who do not have the bad feature).

There is always a trade-off between the two.

Scores must have a high specificity if we assume that it is worse to predict someone is dying, who goes on to survive (because we may falsely opt to withdraw treatments). To achieve satisfactory specificity (say 95%), in practice sensitivity is no better than 33%. That is, we fail to identify most of the people who will die. If we want to identify all those who will die, we will be too gloomy for many who will survive.

In general, we are better at spotting people who will do well, than those who will do badly. Some apparently poor prospects surprise us by recovering.

That said, we must make realistic and humane management plans for dying patients. A deeply unconscious patient a few days after a stroke is not likely to survive. IV hydration may be necessary to temporize, whilst nature takes its course towards death or improvement. 'Primarily palliative' care may be appropriate. But the uncertainty should be acknowledged, and the direction of treatment changed if they improve unexpectedly. This may look like indecision and prevarication, but it is inevitable (and right).

Sometimes doctors and other health professionals will 'get it wrong'— patients will be put through procedures (e.g. feeding tube insertion) or other life-prolonging interventions only to die a few days later, or will survive and remain dependent and miserable. This is not necessarily bad care, but due to the unpredictable nature of the disease.

Some other patients 'fail to thrive' or 'turn their head to the wall' after initial survival. Beware the possibility of severe depression, undiagnosed physical comorbidity, or complications, but consider if these patients too are dying, and offer sympathetic symptom control.

Box 7.1 List of features after stroke associated with increased risk of death

- Unconsciousness.
- Intra-cerebral haemorrhage.
- Total anterior circulation stroke (large MCA infarct).
- Dysphagia.
- Gaze palsy.
- Breathing abnormalities.
- Heart disease.
- Severe comorbidity or pre-existing disability.
- Hyperglycaemia.
- Pyrexia.
- AF.
- Delirium.

Palliative care in stroke—is there a problem?

Many stroke patients die fairly quickly from their strokes, and this will affect the type and nature of palliative care that is appropriate.

The UK Regional Study of Care of the Dying described the experience of symptoms in people dying from stroke (see Box 7.2). Nearly half of people certified as 'dying of a stroke', however, did so a month or more after it occurred. Many symptoms were reported (Table 7.1). Pain, confusion, low mood, and incontinence were particularly common—although we cannot tell which problems were due to the stroke and which were due to comorbidity.

Palliative care is no more of an issue in stroke than other life-threatening conditions, except that stroke has less well-developed support systems than others, cancer in particular. There is less provision for counselling time, and a less developed interface with home care.

Alleviating distressing symptoms is a good thing in its own right. If death is not thought to be imminent, there is a tension between achieving this (with drugs, at least), and an holistic strategy for longer-term health.

Doctors who work with older people are suspicious of symptomatic drug treatments with good reason. All drug treatments carry a burden of side effects, inconvenience, interaction, and compliance problems. Symptoms may be self-limiting, but the drug treatment continued long after it is needed. Geriatricians usually stop as many drugs as they start.

> **Box 7.2 The Regional Study of Care of the Dying**
>
> - Families and carers of 3696 people who died in England in 1990 were surveyed, about 10 months after the death. They were asked to recall problems during the last year of the person's life. Stroke was the main cause of death for 237.
> - Respondents were spouses (20%), siblings or children (37%), other relatives (11%), friends (11%), and professionals (20%). 9% of patients were <65 and 38% over >85 years. 12% died within 24h of the stroke, 18% between a day and a week, and 22% between a week and a month. 11% died at home. 19% spent all of their last year in a hospital, residential home, or nursing home.
> - Respondents reported that hospital doctors and GPs tried hard to control symptoms, but between a quarter and a half were inadequately relieved. 80% felt that care by hospital doctors or nurses was adequate.
>
> *Stroke* 1995; **26**:2242–48.

Table 7.1 Symptoms perceived as problems by carers of people who died from stroke, excluding sudden deaths

	In last month of life (%)	In last year of life (%)
Urinary incontinence	51	56
Pain	42	65
Confusion	41	51
Low mood	33	57
Faecal incontinence	31	38
Poor appetite	29	37
Difficulty breathing	28	37
Constipation	23	46
Poor sleep	22	42
Swallowing problems	20	23
Dry mouth or thirst	20	31
Anxiety	18	26
Pressure sores	17	21
Unpleasant smell	13	16
Nausea or vomiting	12	22
Persistent cough	8	15

Palliative and terminal care

'Palliating' is 'alleviation without curing'. Strictly, this is what happens in most of medicine. It is not non-treatment, or withdrawal of active treatments. Instead, it is a prioritization of treatments with the aim of relieving distress, minimizing burden related to treatment, and restoring what independence, autonomy, and control is possible in the circumstances.

'Terminal care' is the management of patients in whom the advent of death is felt to be certain, and not far off, and for whom medical effort is wholly directed at relief of symptoms, and psychological support of patient and family rather than cure or prolongation of life.

The key principles of palliative medicine are:
- Meticulous management of symptoms.
- Open communication.
- Psychological, emotional, and spiritual support of the patient and of those close to them.

The time frame over which palliative care issues occur stretches from a few hours to several months. Four patterns are seen in stroke care, which result in death:
1. Severe stroke, leading to rapid neurological death.
2. Complications of stroke, e.g. pneumonia, in the early or recovery phase.
3. 'Stroke presentation' of tumour, inoperable abscess, or subdural haematoma.
4. 'Incidental' stroke occurring in someone dying from another condition, such as cancer or severe heart or respiratory failure.

Symptom control

The clinical approach in palliative care has much in common with rehabilitation; problem-orientated and pragmatic, in the face of chronic or progressive illness.

- Write a problem list:
  - Identify each symptom, disability, or problem.
  - Understand its importance (how much does it bother you?) and consequences.
  - Note previous successful and unsuccessful treatments.
- Explain each problem:
  - Understand how each symptom has arisen.
  - If you can't find a cause, guess the most likely one (primary disease process, comorbid disease, iatrogenic or other treatment-related problems?)
  - Are psychological factors or comorbidity exacerbating the problem?
- Treat the treatable:
  - Give the specific treatment if symptoms can be relieved by curing a pathology, such as a chest infection.
  - Think broadly and laterally, e.g. agitation may be caused by pain, urinary retention, hypoxia, drugs, or constipation.
  - Use a treatment which can be expected to address the mechanism of the symptoms if the underlying pathology cannot be cured.
- Assess the effect of the treatment:
  - Best-guess treatment will not work every time.
  - Multiple causes for the one symptom can cause apparent treatment failure. Relief of one symptom may reveal another.
  - Symptoms may change. Progressive diseases will cause new or worsening symptoms over time.
  - Stop drugs if you are not sure they are needed. They can always be restarted.
- Anticipate problems:
  - Opiates always cause constipation, and often cause nausea.
  - Drug withdrawal (opiates, nicotine, alcohol), and commencement (opiates or steroids) can cause agitation.
  - Pressure sores are avoidable.
- Decisions about symptom control fall within the general framework of benefits and burdens, patient choice or best interests, and non-discrimination.
- Table 7.2 gives a list of common symptoms, and some approaches to addressing them. There is a specialist Palliative Care Formulary, which lists some specialized or unlicensed uses of drugs (see ℘ http://www.palliativedrugs.com, which has a searchable symptom list).

Table 7.2 Common (non-pain) symptoms in terminal care

Symptom	Possible causes	Symptomatic treatment
Agitation	Pain, constipation, retention, hypoxia, hypoglycaemia, other metabolic disturbance, anxiety, dementia, delirium (and its causes, including drugs)	Specific cause. Trazodone 50–150mg at night, risperidone 0.5–1mg bd, haloperidol 0.5–10mg bd to 10mg tds, lorazepam 1–2mg bd
Anorexia	Infection, depression, nausea, pain, constipation, denture problems, sore mouth	Dietary measures (small portions, soft consistency, preferences, supplements, alcohol). Can try prednisolone 10–30mg od, megestrol 80–160mg bd
Breathlessness	Heart failure, chronic lung disease, lung or pleural malignancy, pleural effusion, pulmonary embolism, pneumonia, chest deformity, acidosis, anxiety	Specific cause. Explanation. Fan, nebulized bronchodilator; Opiates ± lorazepam, or hyoscine butylbromide (for retained secretions)
Constipation	Immobility, dehydration, drugs, anorexia, hypercalcaemia	Senna 15–30mg, docusate 200mg bd, picosulfate 5–10mg, or movicol 1–8 sachets/day, co-danthramer 2 capsules once at night (increasing up to tds). Consider glycerin suppositories, or enemas
Drooling	Dysphagia, facial weakness	Ipatropium bromide (atrovent) inhaler, transdermal hyoscine hydrobromide or glycopyrronium 200–400mcg tds PO
Faecal incontinence	Impaction with overflow, disinhibited colon, diarrhoeal disease, laxatives and other drugs, immobility, and communication problems	Clear bowels (abdominal X-ray to assess). Pads, prompted toileting, faecal collecting bags. Loperamide/enemas bowel regimen if planning discharge
Fitting	Stroke, tumour, infection, uraemia, hyponatraemia, hypoglycaemia	Oral (or nasogastric) valproate, IV phenytoin, rectal carbamazepine, SC midazolam infusion (20–40mg/24h)
Insomnia	Pain, noise, depression, nocturia	Specific cause. Temazepam, trazodone, or amitriptyline

Nausea	Drugs (especially opiates), constipation, raised intracranial pressure, medullary stroke, hypercalcaemia, uraemia, gastric or bowel stasis or obstruction, disseminated malignancy	Consult a specialist text for logical drug choices. Metoclopramide, cyclizine, haloperidol, levomepromazine, hyoscine, ondansetron, or combinations. Sometimes dexamethasone or benzodiazepines
Sore mouth	Dehydration, mouth breathing, candidiasis, aphthous ulcers, denture problems, gingivitis	Chlorhexidine mouth wash, pineapple chunks, nystatin or fluconazole for candida, buccal analgesics (benzydamine, bonjela), triamcinolone in orabase for ulcers
Urinary incontinence	Unstable bladder, incomplete emptying/retention, inability to communicate or move	Prompted voiding, pads, sheath, intermittent or indwelling catheter

Pain management

- Assess each pain. There may be more than one.
- Unrelieved pain is intensified by insomnia, depression, anxiety, social isolation, and hopelessness. Consider antidepressants as adjuvants to analgesics.
- Get control of the pain quickly. Which drug you choose depends on initial severity. Use oral or SC morphine or diamorphine if necessary, and then decide on a regular regimen.
- Give analgesics regularly for constant or recurring pain. Prescribe short-acting, as-required, medication for acute exacerbations ('break-through pain') in spite of regular analgesia.
- Always give paracetamol 1g qds. This may be sufficient to control the pain, if not it will reduce the requirement for stronger and more toxic drugs.
- Next add a 'weak opiate'. Dihydrocodeine is poorly tolerated by elderly people (delirium, drowsiness, nausea, constipation, malaise). Tramadol (50–100mg qds) is often better, but can also cause delirium and constipation. Low-dose buprenorphine transdermal patches (5–20mcg/h) can be helpful. Non-steroidal anti-inflammatory drugs (ibuprofen 400mg tds, diclofenac 50mg tds) if there is likely an inflammatory component.
- If this is insufficient, use morphine or diamorphine.
- All patients on strong opiates become constipated—prescribe senna 2 tablets (15mg) od or bd plus sodium docusate 200mg bd, or co-danthramer, initially 2 capsules at night. Laxatives may need to be given several times a day.
- 30–50% of patients on strong opiates get nausea, but it is transient (give cyclizine 50mg tds or metoclopramide 10mg tds for first week). Drowsiness is also usually transient (few days). Dry mouth is common. Other opiate-induced problems include hallucinations (try a different opiate, or use haloperidol), vivid dreams, myoclonus (use clonazepam), gastric stasis, and itch.
- Tolerance is a minor problem. Addiction is defined as an overpowering drive to take a drug for its psychological effects, associated with behaviours such as drug seeking, escalating doses, loss of social control, and neglect of personal hygiene. Addiction does not occur with drugs taken for pain control, and patients can be reassured of this.
- Alternative opiates are higher dose transdermal buprenorphine (35mcg/h), or fentanyl patches (12–25mcg/h applied for 3 days at a time, steady state in 12–24h, less constipating than morphine, but the smallest patch starts at a high dose for frail elderly people); oxycodone (less drowsiness and delirium, fewer dreams and hallucinations, available rectally), and hydromorphone (less drowsiness).
- For neuropathic (burning or shooting quality, allodynia—unpleasant sensation of normal stimuli, usually with altered tactile sensation), or central poststroke pain, try pregabalin (50mg bd to 150mg bd) and / or amitriptyline (25–100mg at night). Other drugs or acupuncture may work, but are difficult to use—seek specialist help. CPSP is always difficult to treat.

- Pains that respond poorly or only partly to opiates include:
  - Neuropathic pain.
  - Bone pain (add a non-steroidal anti-inflammatory drug, radiotherapy).
  - Raised intracranial pressure (use dexamethasone, radiotherapy).
  - Tension headache (paracetamol, non-steroidal anti-inflammatory drugs).
  - Muscle cramp.

Routes of drug administration

- The oral route is often not available because dying stroke patients are either drowsy or unable to swallow.
- Rectal absorption is good for paracetamol, diclofenac, domperidone, and carbamazepine.
- Transdermal preparations for fentanyl, buprenorphine and hyoscine hydrobromide (1mg/72h).
- Transmucosal lorazepam, prochlorperazine, and phenazocin are available.
- SC metoclopramide, cyclizine, hyoscine butylbromide, haloperidol, and diamorphine can be given (use a 22G butterfly needle).
- Syringe drivers are useful, especially in the agonal (immediately pre-death) phase.

Does symptom control hasten death?

- Palliative care intends neither to hasten nor postpone death.
- Good symptom control may extend rather than shorten life.
- If symptom control measures do shorten life, this is permissible in English law if the intention is relief of suffering, rather than expediting death (the principle of double effect, R v Bodkin Adams 1957—an act which is foreseen to have both good and bad effects is legitimate, provided the act itself is good or at least neutral, the good effect is not caused by the bad effect, and the bad is proportionate to the good).
- Motivation and proportionality are hard to judge. If the sole reason for doing something is to hasten death it is both illegal and wrong.

The last few days of life

- Encourage participation by the patient's family and friends, in decision making and practical care, according to views and wishes.
- Reassess needs. Look for non-verbal clues of distress (agitation, grimacing, groaning), examine possible sites of pain (mouth, ears, heels).
- Treat distressing symptoms, and stop all other medication. Pain can always be controlled, but sometimes at the cost of drowsiness or continual sleep.
  - Use morphine or diamorphine SC, intermittently or by syringe driver. If the patient has not had opiates before start with diamorphine 5–10mg/24h. If opiates have been used before, the dose will depend on previous doses, response, body build, and renal function.
  - Other drugs can be added to a syringe driver according to the clinical situation, and may include:
    ○ haloperidol (initially 2.5mg/24h) for nausea or agitation.
    ○ midazolam (initially 10mg/24h) for anxiety or fitting.
    ○ hyoscine butylbromide (60mg/24h) for retained respiratory secretions.
  - Levomepromazine (start at 5–25mg/24h), is a powerful antiemetic and sedative, which may also be analgesic, and can be given SC. Sedation is usual with doses >50mg/day.
- Prescribe as required medication for anticipated symptoms—agitation, anxiety, pain, convulsions, noisy respiratory secretions.
- Stop routine observations and investigations unless there is a specific problem to solve, which enhances comfort.
- Dry mouth is caused by mouth breathing, drugs, and/or poor fluid intake. Parenteral fluids are rarely needed. Dehydration is not painful and patients rarely complain of thirst. Continued hydration may increase the distress of dying. Use local measures to relieve dry mouth. These must be done regularly and assiduously. Relatives can usefully help in doing this.
- If someone is dying and unable to swallow safely, they should not be denied access to oral fluids (or food if they ask for it). Whilst it is legal to withdraw IV or tube hydration, it is illegal to deny oral fluids to someone who wants them. Clearly if distressing choking occurs, the patient may revise their wishes, but staff should not otherwise worry about the risk of aspiration.
- Continue skin care and containment of incontinence—use a sheath, pads, or a catheter if necessary.
- Assess relatives' needs.
- Consider discharge home.
- An end of life care pathway (e.g. Liverpool Care Pathway; ✍ http://www.mcpcil.org.uk/liverpool-care-pathway/) can be useful to prompt assessments, management changes and clinical reviews, using explicit documentation designed for the purpose. But note that the 'criteria for use' apply to many stroke patients who are not dying.

If the patient is unconscious, or nearly so, and shows no signs of distress, some treatments which are neutral in terms of benefit or harm to the patients can be justified if they help relieve distress in relatives. Examples include a 'cosmetic' SC fluid infusion, hyoscine for excessive respiratory secretions, diamorphine or haloperidol for agitation or restlessness. Beware features such as grimacing or agitation that may indicate under-treatment.

Psychological support—patients and families

- Psychological assessment and management after a stroke is all the more difficult because of confusion, drowsiness, and aphasia, which are common in patients with severe strokes. In many cases there will be no meaningful verbal communication between the patient and staff.
- By definition, an unconscious patient has no distressing symptoms, physical or psychological. But watch for clues that this is not the case if consciousness is depressed but not completely lost.
- A drowsy patient who is not agitated probably has no distress, but it is difficult to be sure. Hearing is said to be the last of the senses to be lost. Assume that drowsy patients can hear, and welcome attention and company. Don't talk as if they are not there. Reassure relatives that their presence is helpful, even when they seem to be getting little response in return. Encourage staff not to neglect patients because routine observations have been stopped.
- Communication is the cornerstone of effective psychological support. This comprises listening and talking. Good communication saves time, is more satisfying, and less stressful. Tailor the giving of information to the wishes and understanding of the recipient, especially that involving bad news.
- Be empathetic. Empathy is putting yourself in someone else's shoes. If we have not been in a similar situation ourselves, we must use our imaginations. People differ one from another, so not everyone's feelings and emotions will be the same as your own. Recognize both the distress of dying or seeing a close relative die, and of being in a strange and disempowering environment (hospital).
- Most people fear death. But many older people are remarkably philosophical about it, realize that lifespan is not infinite, and will have seen contemporaries die. If the patient is able to engage, you can assume that they will have thought about their own death in general terms. Many dying patients are aware of what is happening (see Table 7.3). Most understand and accept. However, in the Regional Study of Care of the Dying, patients dying with stroke were more likely to have to work this out for themselves than were cancer patients (who were more often told by professionals). This means that either the professionals did not know, or were reluctant to share the information.
- Some patients use the psychological defence of denial. If this is protective allow it to continue. If it is creating problems it may need to be challenged. Patients or relatives may insist on non-disclosure of the truth to the other party. This is usually counter-productive. Ask them why? Explanations include previous bad experience, protecting themselves, or a mutual wish to avoid distress. Ask what they know already. It is often more than you think. Isolation, mistrust, and lack of knowledge increase fear and anxiety. Ultimately, the doctor's first duty is to the patient who has a right to know. Be aware of the specific parietal lobe deficit of anosognosia (denial of having a stroke), which is 'neurological' rather than psychological.

Table 7.3 Awareness that the patient was going to die in the Regional Study of Care of the Dying (data from Addington-Hall J. In *Managing Terminal Illness* (eds. G Ford and I Lewin), Royal College of Physicians of London, 1996)

		Stroke %	Heart disease %	Cancer %
Patients	Knew	40	49	76
	Did not know	35	39	16
	Not known	25	12	8
Carers	Knew	57	37	77
	Half knew	22	22	13
	Did not know	22	41	11
Worked it out for themselves	Patients	80	81	42
	Carers	36	42	20

- Ignorance can cause fear. Try to find out what the patient or relatives fear most:
  - Uncontrolled pain is rare.
  - Fear of inappropriate discharge from hospital, or moving between different wards, is common in a health service pressed for bed capacity. If death is likely within a week or two, patients and relatives should be reassured that they should not be moved unless they want to (e.g. to go home, or to a more conveniently located nursing home). Terminally ill patients in the British NHS have a right not to be discharged.
  - If death is less imminent, fear of dependency, confusion, or incontinence may be allayed by convincing practical plans.
  - Fear of overintervention and artificial prolongation of the end of life should be allayed by reassurance.
  - How the family will cope, and finances, are common fears. Most are lessened by being shared even if not fully resolved.
- Anxiety and depression are almost inevitable in dying patients who are alert and cognitively unimpaired. However, in the context of stroke, this is rarely the case.
- Patients with aphasia have the added burden of frustration and the inability to express their feelings or sometimes to understand information given to them.
- Allow expression of emotion, and make room for cultural and religious beliefs or practices which you may not share or feel comfortable with.

- Create a sense of partnership in decision making and care giving. Aim for continuity of care. Anything which enables participation, independence, and a sense of control is good.
- Saying 'don't worry' is unhelpful. Reassurance without explanation is unconvincing and can increase anxiety. A counselling approach is better but time consuming. Get the patient or relatives to state what the problems are, and with the help of some technical explanation, what the possible solutions are. The trick is to give at least the impression of having time to take on problems, which you can do by listening to problems and being sympathetic to them.
- Care of dying people is emotionally costly for staff. Team support is important. You must have confidence in your colleagues (of any discipline) and them in you, and be ready to ask their advice.
- Don't exclude young children. Everyone will want to protect them from distress, but they are perceptive, and exclusion and isolation in the long-run makes things worse.
- Spiritual pain is rather alien to our current way of thinking about life. Death raises questions of life and its meaning, feelings of guilt and failure about the past, things left undone, failed relationships. Life may seem meaningless. Patients and relatives may be thinking in these terms even if you are not. Acknowledge them if the opportunity arises.

Bereavement

'Bereavement' describes both the experience of grieving, and the time period during which it occurs. Grieving is the feeling of sorrow, and other emotional reactions, after a loss. This is usually seen in its most intense form after a death, but may be seen as a response to other losses after a stroke—including loss of health, function, body image, roles, interests, and relationships.

People respond to loss in different ways. Sometimes this is unpredictable and unexpected—to everyone, the person themselves, those around them, and staff, including yourself. Understanding the process can help them and us. But don't expect to understand everything, nor for reactions to be logical or 'reasonable'. Sometimes the process may seem alien or embarrassing (such as prayers or high levels of visibly expressed emotion), and sometimes it will get personal (anger and complaints directed against staff). You just have to accept this as part of the job. Try to be tolerant and sympathetic, even if that is not how you feel.

Reaction to a death depends in part on what has gone before:
• Sudden unexpected death. There is no preparation, or anticipation, and in general the impact on surviving relatives will be more severe and disruptive.
• Death in the week or two after a stroke. Often there is a period of uncertainty before death, about survival and the prospect of severe disability, and the balance between life-sustaining supportive medical care and terminal symptom control. But this time allows families some time to adjust to the prospect of loss ('anticipatory grief').
• Death from a late complication, recurrence, or other vascular disease—the initial shock and threat to life will have been experienced, and, to some extent, adjusted to.

Other important contributors include:
• The personality and personality traits of the grieving person.
• Their personal coping abilities and things that compromise them, such as physical and mental illness.
• Things that enhance coping, including family and social support (including cultural and religious influences).
• The nature, characteristics, and closeness of the relationship with the deceased person.
• Their previous experiences of grieving.

Bereavement can bring overwhelming physical and emotional distress, and be frightening and bewildering. Psychological reactions can include:
• Anger.
• Guilt.
• Anxiety.
• Sadness.
• Despair.
• Crying.

Physical responses include:
- Fatigue.
- Sleep disturbance.
- Loss of appetite.
- Bodily symptoms.

Guilt may include the feeling that 'everything possible was not done'. Anger can easily be directed at medical and nursing staff, especially if relatives were dissatisfied with, or misunderstood, some aspect of care. Hence an important preventative function is served by good, sympathetic, communicative, terminal care.

There are a number of theories about grieving. Kubler-Ross's ground-breaking idea that grieving people work through a number of stages (numbness, denial, searching, anger, resolution), is no longer thought to be adequate. Phases of grief are recognized, but people may move back and forward through them.

They include:
- Shock and numbness—difficulty in taking in information about the death (so it may need to be repeated; and the need for the grieving person to rehearse the details is not endlessly going on about the death).
- Yearning and searching—intense separation anxiety, and disregard of the reality of the loss, which leads to the need to search for the missing person, with inevitable disappointment.
- Disorganization and despair—with depression, distractibility and poor concentration, and difficulty planning for the future.
- Reorganization and recovery.

A bereaved person eventually needs to adapt and reintegrate into the world. This involves:
- Accepting the reality of the loss.
- Experiencing, expressing, and resolving the physical and emotional distress of loss.
- Adjustment to the environment from which the person is missing.
- Redirecting the emotional energy previously invested in the person who died.
- Forming new relationships.

Over a few months the symptoms fade. Health professionals need to recognize delayed, inhibited, or chronic grief. Of course, by this time events are probably far removed from the hospital stroke ward, but you may come across bereaved people in other contexts, and sometime repercussions come late (requests to discuss what happened, complaints).

A third of bereaved spouses develop significant physical or mental health problems, and are twice as likely as expected to die in the following year. Health consequences are worse if the death is of a young person, if there are low levels of trust, a previous history of psychiatric disease, a perceived lack of support or understanding, or if the relationship with the deceased was overdependant.

Information can be especially short when the death is unexpected. Bereavement support services are usually available locally.

Summary

1. Many stroke patients die, often days to weeks after hospital admission. For some a palliative care approach is appropriate, either alone or in tandem with supportive management.

2. Although several prognostic markers have been identified after stroke, and several prognostic scores have been developed, none is accurate enough to be very useful in clinical stroke management. However, patients who are unconscious several days after a stroke are unlikely to survive.

3. Carers of patients dying of a stroke report many distressing symptoms, resulting either from the stroke itself, or from comorbid disease.

4. Palliation is the alleviation of symptoms without cure. Palliative care is the prioritization of treatments with the aim of relieving distress, minimizing burden related to treatment, and restoring what independence, autonomy, and control is possible in the circumstances.

5. Multiple and complex symptoms and problems must be meticulously assessed, explained, and whatever curative or palliative treatment is possible used to relieve them.

6. A considerable body of expertise exists in the control of pain and other distressing symptoms.

7. Open explanation and communication is vital, but is often difficult in dying stroke patients, who may be drowsy, aphasic, or confused.

8. Allowing family to be involved in decision making and delivering practical care is both useful for the patient (and staff) and therapeutic for themselves.

9. Anticipate, identify, and address fears.

10. Grieving is an intense emotional and physical experience. It is often unpredictable, and needs to be managed with tolerance and sympathy, even when reactions appear unreasonable.

Chapter 8

Rehabilitation

What is rehabilitation?

A dictionary definition is: 'a restoration to rights or former abilities'. Rehabilitation is more a philosophy than a treatment, with a focus on function and solving practical problems.

There are three elements:
- Reablement—restoration of function, taking advantage of spontaneous recovery, avoiding complications, learning new skills, and making use of aids and appliances.
- Resettlement—the adaptation of the environment to suit the abilities of the person concerned, and maximize their participation.
- Readjustment—psychological adaptation, changes in goals and ambitions, re-establishing esteem, and fulfilment.

And two broad aims:
- To maximize functional ability.
- To increase the number of options that patients and their families have over eventual discharge—which often means making possible a home discharge where the alternative would have been institutional care.

How to approach rehabilitation

- Make a problem list. Identify, break down, and understand problems. This requires assessment by medical, nursing, and therapy disciplines, including a thorough review of the casenotes, discussion with the patient about what is happening, what they understand and what they want, and consultation with family or other carers.
- Set goals—these can be:
  - 'High-level goals', where you eventually want to get (e.g. independence walking, discharge home).
  - 'Intermediate goals', things that need to be achieved on the way to the higher-level goals (such as standing, or weight transference between legs).
- Intervene therapeutically.
- Review progress, revise the problem list, and repeat the cycle until all goals are met, or a plateau is reached, when we assume that maximum ability has been achieved.
- Make plans to deal with, or compensate for, any remaining problems.
- Continually reconsider the most appropriate location for rehabilitation, and commence discharge planning.

Convene an early meeting with family, including the patient if he or she is able. Discuss:
- What they have already been told and what they already know.
- Previous abilities, problems, and support.
- The diagnosis and its effects, especially on current abilities.
- Their expectations.
- The likely prognosis.
- Future options:
  - Keep all options open for as long as possible. Don't make any assumptions (e.g. that institutional discharge will be inevitable).
  - The likely duration of recovery and rehabilitation.
  - Broach the possibility of institutional discharge if it looks likely. Suggest that family members visit a few care homes (in the UK the website of the Care Quality Commission [🖰 www.cqc.org.uk] is a good place to start). This enables future discussions to be better informed, and starts the process of finding a suitable home.

If the patient was previously living in a care home, useful information about previous abilities and goals (e.g. what abilities are required to enable a return to the previous home) can be gained by telephoning the home.

Problems

(See Table 8.1.)
'Problems' (in the problem list) can be:

- A risk factor or predisposition (e.g. smoking).
- Diagnoses or complications.
- Abnormalities of body structure or function (impairment).
- An inability to perform tasks or activities (sometimes called 'disabilities').
- Restricted participation—problems at the level of the person in a physical and social environment.

The relationship between these, and the place of different interventions and barriers can be seen from Fig. 8.1. If any element is missing, opportunities to improve functioning may be missed.

A comprehensive assessment is essential to avoid difficulties and delays later on. Some commonly-occurring issues need specific plans, some of which may be ongoing from earlier in the admission (Box 8.1).

Table 8.1 Impairment, activity limitations, and participation restrictions

Impairments	Activity limitations/ disabilities	Participation restrictions
• Poor sitting balance	• Sitting	• Inability to get where needed or desired
• Limb weakness	• Transferring	
• Spasticity/contractures	• Walking	• Loss of independence—need for help with daily activities
• Hemianopia	• Stair climbing	
• Aphasia	• Continence	• Inability to undertake occupation and responsibilities—employment, leisure, domestic
• Visuospatial problems/ neglect	• Toilet use	
• Visual field defect	• Dressing	
• Poor visual acuity	• Feeding	
• Depression/anxiety	• Kitchen skills	• Poor awareness of surroundings
• Lack of confidence or motivation	• Washing, bathing, showering	• Inability to sustain social relationships
• Poor memory, concentration, judgement, problem solving	• Behavioural disturbance	• Participation in civic responsibilities
	• Communication problems	
• Detrusor instability		
• Polyuria		
• Breathlessness		
• Pain (joints, central)		
• Deafness		

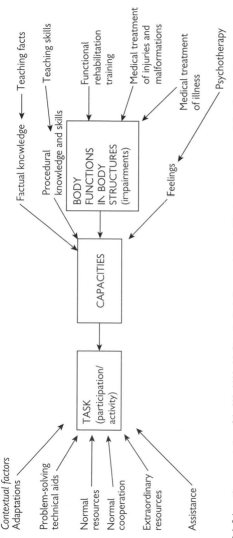

Fig. 8.1 Schematic representation of the World Health Organization's framework for rehabilitation—the *International Classification of Functioning, Disability and Health* (ICF). The aim is to maximize activity and participation. Arrows represent necessary conditions. Devised by Dr Tormod Jaksholt.

Box 8.1 Multidisciplinary rehabilitation headings

- Swallow and nutrition.
- Pressure areas, wound care.
- Positioning, spasticity prevention and management.
- Upper limb function.
- Movement and mobility.
- Standing/transfers/walking.
- Safety/falls.
- Lower urinary tract symptoms and continence.
- Bowels and faecal continence.
- Mood and psychological care.
- Sleep.
- Cognition and perception.
- Communication.
- Washing and dressing.
- Bathing.
- Kitchen skills.
- Home situation and capabilities prior to admission.
- Medication management.
- Secondary prevention and lifestyle modification.
- Discharge planning.

Rehabilitation nursing

Rehabilitation nursing may be the single most important element of a rehabilitation unit, requiring flexibility and fine judgement. It involves:

- Using opportunities during daily care to undertake functional activities (getting up, toileting, dressing, walking to the day room or to meals).
- The progressive withdrawal of support as independence and confidence are regained.

This is achieved through:

- Practice of skills or approaches learnt with specialist rehabilitation therapists, and avoidance of poor positioning or inappropriate activities ('the 24-h approach').
- The building of stamina, fitness, and confidence through physical activity.
- Avoidance of complications (pressure sores, joint contractures, venous thrombosis, aspiration, falls).
- Making specialist assessments and management plans for continence and wound care.
- Providing detailed feedback on day-to-day performance.
- Helping to formulate, and working towards, defined goals.
- Providing sufficient help to ensure 'personal maintenance' (hygiene, nutrition, freedom from falls and other danger).
- Being aware of general health, and the ability to react appropriately in a medical crisis.
- Helping to promote psychological adjustment (listening, advising, encouraging a positive outlook).
- Being aware of, and managing, patients' and relatives' expectations, in particular where this is manifest as dysfunctional illness behaviour (such as overdependency or overprotectiveness), or overoptimistic goals. Some patients expect to be 'cared for' when they should be learning independence.

Teamwork

- A team is a group of people working together with a common purpose.
- Teams achieve more than individuals working in isolation.
- Each team member should know what they bring to the team, their skills and limitations, and what they are responsible for. Doctors in particular, should not forget that it is their job to get the general medicine right (diagnosis, drug therapy, referral to other specialists).
- Team members should know what other members do. There will be some overlap, but unnecessary replication should be avoided (Table 8.2).
- The team should follow the same approach and strategy 24h a day, regardless of which discipline they are from.
- Communication is essential, usually via weekly team meetings, when patients are systematically reviewed for problems, abilities, progress towards goals, and when new goals are set and discharge planning undertaken.
- Each involved team member needs to contribute to meetings—and be helped to do so if reticent.
- An objective record of disabilities should be kept, by using standardized scales, or free text.
- Records should be shared or easily accessible to all team members.
- Leadership of healthcare teams tends to be quite informal—meetings need chairing or directing, but decisions are a matter of consensus, and delegation requires persuasion rather than giving orders (see Box 8.2).

Box 8.2 Leadership and team working

Leaders
- Leaders do not just give orders, but enable people to do their jobs better.
- Team members enable their leaders to lead, because it is in their interests, makes it easier for them to do their own jobs, and helps to achieve a worthwhile common goal.

Leadership functions
- Helping set goals.
- Integrating information.
- Maintaining momentum.
- Making or confirming decisions.
- Developing a vision, identifying new opportunities.

Team working needs
- Clear and agreed roles and duties.
- Equal commitment.
- Shared responsibility.
- Identification and use of individuals' strengths.
- Clear communication and sharing of information.
- Honest, constructive feedback, including thanks and praise.
- Mutual support (e.g. when things go wrong).

Table 8.2 Who does what? Roles of different members of the multi-disciplinary stroke team

Who?	What?
Nurses	Observation, hygiene, basic nutrition, pressure area care, medication supervision, continence management, counselling, primary information point for family, continuity, practice of activities of daily living skills, 24-h approach, discharge planning
Physiotherapists	Assessment and training of motor function, management of abnormal muscle tone and shoulder pain, remediation of mobility disabilities (including trunk control, bed mobility, transfers, walking, and stairs). Other specialist functions may include advice on orthoses, clearing secretions from the lungs, and teaching pelvic floor exercises
Occupational therapists	Assessment and training in personal and domestic activities of daily living, assessment of perceptual abnormalities (neglect, visuospatial problems), apraxias and cognition, seating and wheelchair assessment, home assessment visits, advising on and provision of aids and adaptations. Limb splinting
Speech and language therapists	Assessment and management of neurogenic dysphagia. Assessment and treatment of receptive and expressive language function. Communication training. Provision of communication aids. Advising families and other staff on communication. Support for aphasic patients and their families
Doctors	Compiling comprehensive medical formulation—diagnosis, including comorbidity, risk factors, complications. Medical therapy and necessary specialist referral. Depending on local arrangements, coordination and overview, communication with patients and families
Dieticians	Assessment of nutritional needs, and recommendations on specialist diets (including cholesterol and weight reduction). Planning of tube feeding regimens
Clinical (neuro) psychologists	Assessment of cognitive impairments, perceptual disorders, executive functions (planning, decision making), mood disorders, anxiety, adjustment reactions, and emotionalism. Explanation to patients, carers, and clinical staff. Direct clinical interventions include cognitive retraining, group or individual psychotherapy, relaxation, and cognitive behavioural therapy. Supportive counselling and groups for carers
Social workers	Mainly discharge planning: need for home care support services, meals at home, day centres, institutional care, including respite care. Advice and assessment for financial benefits and institutional care funding. Assessment of carer needs. Also may help with suspected abuse, debt counselling, guardianship, Deprivation of Liberty Safeguards and Mental Health Act orders

Monitoring progress

Progress is best monitored by assessing disability (activity limitation). Three key dimensions are:

- Mobility—transfers, walking, stability and falls, getting to the toilet, stairs, wheelchair use. Include distance achieved, and extent of help and aids required (e.g. walks 20 metres with a wheeled Zimmer frame plus one person). Formal scores such as the Rivermead mobility assessment (see 📖 Appendix 11, p.341) may be used by physiotherapists.
- Continence—and other practical elimination issues such as constipation, nocturia, and urinary urgency.
- Behaviour—usually in the context of dementia or a difficult premorbid personality trait, but also mood, motivation, engagement, and passivity.

Other aspects such as dressing, and kitchen skills, should be added at the appropriate stage of rehabilitation.

In hospital, a standardized activities of daily living (ADL) scale (e.g. Barthel Index—see 📖 Appendix 12, p.342) can be used. Ensure sufficient annotation to record the presumed mechanism of outstanding problems. Is the transfer difficulty due to weakness, pain, dizziness, or fear? This may prompt a medical review.

Once home, a wider range of activities should be considered, including driving or use of public transport, domestic tasks, and shopping.

Prognostication and prediction—trajectories of recovery

Trying to anticipate future progress and outcome is required for two reasons:
- Goal setting, and giving of prognostic information.
- To chart recovery and detect deviations, which might indicate complications or the need for reassessment.

Anticipated rate of recovery depends on initial severity. The Copenhagen Stroke Study (Box 8.3) provided detailed weekly information on recovery patterns:
- Recovery in neurological impairments preceded recovery in functional abilities by about 2 weeks.
- Overall, 80% of surviving patients had reached their best ADL function within 6 weeks of stroke onset, and 95% within 12.5 weeks.
- Recovery in both impairments and disabilities was most rapid in the *least* badly affected patients (Scandinavian Stroke Score, SSS 45–58). Maximum recovery occurred by 8.5 weeks.
- Moderately affected patients (SSS 30–44) had maximum recovery by 13 weeks.
- Severely affected patients (SSS 15–29) had maximum recovery by 17 weeks.
- The most severely affected patients (SSS <15) did not reach a plateau until 20 weeks.

Box 8.3 Recovery patterns: the Copenhagen Stroke Study

- 1197 hospital-admitted acute stroke patients were assessed weekly using the Barthel Index and SSS.
- Evaluation continued until death or discharge, and was repeated 6 months poststroke.
- Initial severity, based on SSS score, was:
  - 19% very severe (SSS <15).
  - 14% severe (SSS 15–29).
  - 26% moderate (SSS 30–44).
  - 41% mild (SSS 45–58).
- Neurological impairment after 6 months (amongst survivors):
  - 11% had severe or very severe deficits.
  - 11% had moderate deficits.
  - 47% had mild deficits.
  - 31% had no or only very mild deficits.

Archives of Physical Medicine and Rehabilitation 1995; **76**:27–32; 399–405; and 406–12.

Caveats

- Do not jump to early conclusions. Some patients regain functional capacities after 6 months—especially, but not exclusively, younger patients.
- Inform patients realistically about the chances of recovery, and negotiate therapy goals. If goals seem overambitious, agree to a period of assessment, or set an intermediate goal that must be achieved in order to reach the more ambitious one. Plans can then be remade if things are going better than expected.

Recovery of motor function can be charted in terms of basic functional tasks ('milestones') agreed by physiotherapists to be important, and which can be assessed very reliably. Table 8.3 illustrates recovery in a series of 368 stroke patients referred for physiotherapy, who survived 8 weeks. This gives a good impression of the rate of recovery in hospital-admitted patients with stroke which compromises functional ability.

Table 8.3 Motor recovery in 368 patients who survived to 8 weeks. Patients were referred within 10 days of their strokes, age range 42–89 years. Items were scored by physiotherapists as able/unable. (Reproduced with permission from Partridge CJ, Johnston M, and Edwards S. Recovery from physical disability after stroke: normal patterns as a basis for evaluation. *Lancet 1987*; i:373–5. Copyright Elsevier (1987).)

Task	% achieving task						
	Referral	1 week	2 weeks	4 weeks	6 weeks	8 weeks
Gross body movements							
Lying, turn head	91	98	99	99	99	99
Maintain sitting balance 2min	59	76	86	91	92	92
Lying, roll onto side	58	73	82	86	89	89
Get up from lying	35	53	64	70	73	76
Stand up to free standing	29	43	52	63	66	71
Transfer bed-chair	27	45	55	63	67	71
2 steps forwards	23	39	48	56	61	66
2 steps backwards	18	33	44	52	57	61
Independent walking inside	14	27	38	45	49	53
Arm movements							
Sitting, clasp and unclasp affected hand	33	47	54	57	60	63
Sitting, place unaffected hand to mouth	27	38	44	49	52	54
Lying, hold arm in elevated position	25	39	45	52	56	56

Mobility

Loss of mobility is fundamental to many of the problems faced in rehabilitation. Mobility disability accounts for at least half of the variation in disability in other areas (if you are immobile, maintaining continence, dressing, kitchen skills, and occupation are difficult).

Impairments contributing to mobility problems include:
- Muscle weakness.
- Balance problems, dizziness, or postural instability.
- Neglect.
- Hemianopia and visual acuity problems.
- Joint instability, contractures, and pain.
- Heel sores.
- Breathlessness.
- Anxiety.
- Psychomotor retardation.
- Advanced dementia.

Each impairment needs identifying, explaining, and treating insofar as is possible. Ask the question 'what is preventing mobility?' Answering requires communication between medical, nursing, and therapy staff.

Most of the recovery in motor impairment is spontaneous. The task of rehabilitation is to:
- Facilitate or enhance this process as much as possible.
- To take advantage of recovery by translating it into useful functions.
- To avoid setbacks caused by complications.

Neurophysiotherapy aims to maximize motor function, reduce abnormal muscle tone, promote symmetricality, and teach normal movement patterns. Early standing is used to establish trunk control. Transferring techniques, and the safe use of mobility aids are also taught. Much therapy is based on neurophysiological theory. Expertise in managing neurological conditions is important, but at least some of the treatment can be delivered by supervised assistants. There is no strong evidence to support the superiority of any one therapy school. More intensive treatment helps, but the optimum intensity is uncertain, and many stroke patients fatigue quickly or otherwise lack stamina. 'Maximum tolerated daily duration and intensity' is the target, but is a vague guideline. Benefit may vary by subgroup, for example, greater benefit for more intensive therapy amongst less severely affected patients.

Some patients benefit from use of specific techniques in addition to conventional physiotherapy, including:
- Partial body weight supported treadmill training: patients with mild to moderate severity stroke can benefit from gait training using a treadmill, with a proportion of bodyweight supported using a harness or sling. This allows repetition of symmetrical movements.
- Constraint-induced movement therapy (CIMT): for patients in the subacute phase with at least some active movement of the arm, constraint-induced therapy can help. This is a standardized treatment based on repetitive task practice using the affected limb, with feedback from a

therapist and 'behavioural shaping' (correction), whilst restraining the unaffected side for 90% of waking hours. Patients must have at least 20 degrees of active wrist extension, 10 degrees of active finger extension, and no significant sensory or cognitive limitation. No more than about 20% of patients are suitable. Therapy is for 6–8h a day for at least 2 weeks (Box 8.4).

- Functional electrical stimulation. This uses an electrical stimulus to make a muscle contract. In general, electrical stimulation alone is not an effective way of strengthening muscles, but can be used to augment a weak self-initiated movement. There are anecdotal reports of improved tone and function. One application assists gait by stimulating tibialis anterior (on the affected side) allowing the foot to dorsiflex as the leg is swung through, stopping it from dragging or catching. Other applications have included reducing shoulder subluxation, and improving wrist and knee extension.
- Orthotics and braces. Mainly to correct foot drop or an unstable knee.

'Deconditioning' is the loss of strength, stamina, cardiorespiratory fitness, balance, and confidence that accompanies acute illness and prolonged disability, especially when associated with subnutrition and infection. Fortunately this can be restored with exercise, and repeated practice at every opportunity is important to achieve this (walking to the toilet, to the day room, the therapy gym). Standard rehabilitation probably does not provide adequate aerobic exercise, and those who can tolerate it should be instructed in appropriate methods of achieving progressively more (walking, treadmill, static bicycle).

'Compensation'—using the unaffected limb to overcome limitations imposed by paralysis—is a difficult topic:
- Some attempts at compensation for hemiparesis are dysfunctional—such as overactivity in the unaffected side ('pushing'), and must be avoided or unlearned. This occurs in about 10% of patients, and delays functional recovery by up to a month.
- Later, compensation is adaptive. Half of patients surviving with initial severe upper limb paralysis get no useful recovery, yet half become independent in upper limb functional tasks by compensatory use of the other limb.

Walking aids and wheelchairs
Walking aids are used to help increase mobility by:
- Improving stability and balance.
- Compensating for muscular weakness.
- Building confidence.
- Prevention of falls.
- Assisting weight bearing following injuries of the lower extremities.

Types of walking aids:
- Walking ('Zimmer') frames, with or without wheels (Fig. 8.2).
- Walking sticks (standard, tripod or quadpod/quadstick; Fig. 8.3).
- Crutches.
- Manual, electric, or companion wheelchairs.
- Wheeled shopping trolleys.
- Electric scooters.

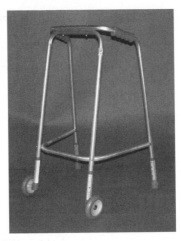

Fig. 8.2 Wheeled Zimmer frame.

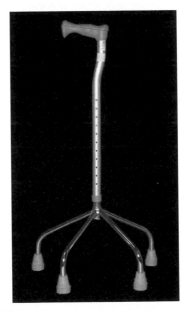

Fig. 8.3 Quad stick.

Box 8.4 Constraint induced movement therapy—EXCITE trial

- 222 participants at nine sites, mean age 62 years, who had had a stroke 3–9 months previously, had 2 weeks of CIMT or usual care. CIMT comprised using a mitt to inhibit use of the unaffected side, whilst performing a repetitive task with the more affected side, for 2h per day. Intervention was at a time when conventional therapy had largely ceased (although about half of each group had some concurrent additional treatment), and further spontaneous recovery was unlikely.
- Outcomes were measured 1, 4, 8, and 12 months later.
- The CIMT group had better performance on the Wolf Motor Function Test, a motor performance test, which contains 15 timed and two strength tasks. Mean time decreased from 19.3s to 9.3s in the active group, compared with a decrease of 24.0s to 17.7s in the control group, representing a difference in change between groups of 34% (95% CI 12–51%).
- The CIMT group also had better performance and in the Motor Activity Log (MAL), a measure of 30 motor-related ADL. In the active group, MAL amount of use, on a 0–5 scale, increased from 1.2 to 2.1 compared with an increase of 1.2 to 1.7 in the control group; a difference in change between groups of 0.43 (95% CI 0.05–0.80). MAL quality of movement, on a 0–5 scale, increased from 1.3 to 2.2 compared with 1.2 to 1.7; a difference in change of 0.48 (95% CI 0.13–0.84).
- The CIMT group achieved a decrease of 19.5 in self-perceived hand function difficulty (Stroke Impact Scale hand domain) vs a decrease of 10.1 for the control group, a difference of 9.4 (95% CI 0.3–18.6).
- Improvements appeared rapidly, persisted throughout follow up, and were still evident after 24 months.

Journal of the American Medical Association 2006; **296**:2095–104.
Lancet Neurology 2008; **7**:33–40.

Physiotherapists are trained to select an appropriate walking device and to 'progress' as recovery occurs:

- A walking stick has to be of the appropriate height (the handle reaching the wrist of the patient while he/she is standing). A 'high stick' may be used (in the unaffected arm) to promote equal weight distribution, as an aid to recovery.
- Further training is needed if the stick is going to be used to climb stairs.
- Tripods and quadpods increase the 'base of support' to provide better stability but they are heavier than standard sticks, and can encourage abnormal movement patterns.
- Crutches are not usually used for patients with stroke but are useful for patients with lower limb injuries.
- Four-legged walking frames (Zimmer frames) must be picked up and advanced with every step, and hence are little use for patients with a paralysed arm. They can be useful for patients with truncal coordination problems (ataxia).
- Wheeled walkers help the patient to walk faster, but at the expense of stability. The addition of wheels assists in pushing the frame forward without lifting.
- For less disabled patients, 3-wheeled delta frames give good speed and manoeuvrability for those who can control them. The patient can change direction without lifting.

Occupational therapists assess the suitability and type of wheelchair and give instruction in their use:

- Wheelchairs may be used indoors though they are often used only for outdoor activity. The companion wheelchair can be folded down to put in a car.
- Motorized wheelchairs and scooters need special assessment.
- Early wheelchair use is controversial. Patients may want the earlier independence (often 'scooting' with the unaffected leg), while therapists worry about the effects on tone and symmetricality.

There is a flourishing private sector selling mobility aids and devices. It may not be easy for patients to get good independent professional advice about the suitability of these products. Some local authorities and voluntary organizations run disability assessment centres where patients can try out aids and get advice.

Stair lifts can be very useful, but a safe transfer on and off, good sitting balance, and freedom from blackouts (e.g. fits) are required.

Outdoor mobility

Outdoor mobility requires balance, confidence, and stamina beyond that needed indoors. The terrain is more challenging, and may be unpredictable. The consequences of falling or otherwise running into trouble are all the more serious:

- One problem is fear—so people perform below the level they are capable of. Encouragement and supervised practice can provide some easy gains, and are most easily delivered in home-based rehabilitation schemes.

- Crowded environments are worrying for people struggling with postural stability. Hospital corridors can be used to start with. Supermarkets are another opportunity for practice, choosing an off-peak time initially.
- Another strategy is to upgrade the walking aid—for example, using a stick indoors and a delta frame outdoors.
- Cars (as driver or passenger) and community disabled transport schemes have the potential to increase participation even when residual problems would make independent outdoor mobility impossible. Practice getting in and out of a car may be required. Accompanied bus or car trips can help to restore confidence leading to eventual independence.
- A mobile phone can alleviate some of the consequences of a fall or other mishap whilst out.

Spasticity

(See also 📖 Spasticity, p.308).

Spasticity is excessive, inappropriate, and involuntary muscle activity resulting in stiffness. Secondary biomechanical factors (muscle short-ening and joint stiffness) are also important. Established spasticity hinders normal movement, and may cause pain, spasms, hyper-reflexia or clonus, and contractures.

Physiotherapy tries to prevent or reduce spasticity, and must commence very early on. Initial changes can occur within a few days of a stroke, and once established are hard to reverse. Achieving some active movement helps prevent spasticity. Splinting of the hand and wrist can help, and may even improve whole arm function, truncal tone, and gait. Patients can be taught methods to lengthen muscles which are at risk of contracture such as calf muscles, forearm muscles, and wrist and finger flexors. Poor posi-tioning, pain (including shoulder pain), constipation, urinary retention, and pressure sores exacerbate spasticity.

Increased tone in the lower limb hinders stepping through of the unaf-fected leg (as it won't 'release'). In the upper limb the increased tone pulls the elbow, wrist, and fingers into flexion. Preventing a completely paralysed hand from contracting is difficult. This can affect dressing, and make hand hygiene impossible. Sometimes a spastic leg (holding the limb in extension) allows weight to be borne for transferring or walking. However, the extended (plantar flexed) foot tends to drag and cause falls. An ankle–foot orthosis (AFO), or functional electrical stimulation (FES) of the dorsiflexors, may help.

Anecdotally, the prevalence of badly contracted limbs and 'circumduc-tion gait' has decreased over recent decades with improvement in therapy techniques and delivery.

Botulinum toxin injections can be used to treat focal spasticity without systemic side effects or inducing weakness. This can be used as early as necessary, but is usually avoided within the first 4–6 weeks, unless:
• Hand contracture is making hygiene difficult.
• Joint range of movement is being lost despite adequate physiotherapy and splinting.
• High tone is causing problems with progressing function (e.g. hamstring spasticity is preventing a standing transfer).

Otherwise drug treatment is generally disappointing. The risk in reducing muscle tone with drugs is that weakness is made worse, and function reduced. Tizanidine, dantrolene, baclofen, and diazepam may be tried but all can cause drowsiness or confusion.

Dexterity

Hand function recovers last and least. Intensive arm training has some effect, but the effect is fairly small. Persisting loss of dexterity, especially in the dominant hand, is a particular problem.

The main therapeutic technique is repeated practice of functional tasks and avoiding disuse. This maintains sensory input, flexibility, and muscle strength.

Shoulder pain

(See also 📖 The affected shoulder, p.58).

Shoulder pain is common, distressing, limits activities—including dressing and walking (Box 8.5)—and may exacerbate arm spasticity.

The mechanism is presumed to be an effect of subluxation due to a weak rotator cuff, but the exact cause is uncertain. Careful handling may help prevent shoulder pain, including limiting passive movement to 30 degrees flexion, extension, or abduction, and avoiding pulling on the affected arm, or lifting under the arm. However, shoulder pain is still seen where best moving and handling practice is undertaken. Sometimes slings or other devices are used to try to prevent shoulder pain, but their effectiveness is uncertain. Patients and relatives should be taught the importance of shoulder care, and to challenge health or social care staff if they are about to perform a potentially damaging manoeuvre.

Assessment and treatment is multidisciplinary, including doctors, physiotherapists, nurses, and occupational therapists. Try to make a diagnosis: comorbid shoulder disease is common (including rotator cuff damage, capsulitis, arthritis). Consult a rheumatologist if this is difficult. Localize the pain, and assess range of movement. Rarely, CPSP is the cause.

Treatment starts with simple and mid-strength analgesia, but this is often insufficient. Intra-articular steroids or acupuncture may be tried. As a last resort use a suprascapular nerve block. Physiotherapy management includes progressive mobilization and muscle activation or strengthening. There is some evidence to support the use of FES.

Box 8.5 Shoulder pain after stroke

- A consecutive series of 416 patients with acute stroke was reviewed at 4 and 16 months. 12% required assistance or a proxy to answer because of aphasia of cognitive problems. 22% has shoulder pain prior to their stroke, and this had little bearing on subsequent experience of pain. After 4 months 16% had died; after 16 months 21% had died.
- 30% experienced new shoulder pain. Pain was rated moderate to severe in 79%.
- 22% had shoulder pain at 4 months, with onset mostly within 2 weeks of stroke.
- At 16 months prevalence was 24%, with half of these developing pain >2 months poststroke. 27% with pain at 4 months no longer had pain. Pain severity was generally less at 16 months. 10% developed pain following a fall.
- Shoulder pain was more common amongst the most severely disabled. The proportion with shoulder pain was 83% among patients with no arm motor function, 50% among patients with reduced function, but only 5% among patients with normal function.
- Pain was more common in those with sensory loss (56% had pain) and clinically defined subluxation (74% had pain). Only 1% had CPSP causing shoulder pain.
- Almost all described pain on movement, 23% pain at rest. 70% had pain on dressing, and in half walking was inhibited by pain. Half were on analgesics.

Stroke 2007; **38**:343–8.

Continence

Continence can make or break the chances of a successful discharge.

Urinary

Half of patients admitted to hospital are initially incontinent of urine.

- About half of these have detrusor hyper-reflexia (an unstable or overactive bladder, one which contracts before it is full and when the patient does not want it to, a failure of inhibition of detrusor contractions).
- Frontal lobe lesions sometimes result in an extreme form of this— urinary precipitancy, where there is no warning at all.
- A quarter have retention.
- The other quarter have normal bladder function (on cystometry). Presumably their problems are due to awareness, communication, immobility, and lack of access of suitable aids (urinals, commodes, or toilets).

In each case the abnormality may be due to the stroke or comorbid pathology:

- 20% of stroke patients have continence problems before their stroke.
- 20% of people over 70 have detrusor instability in the absence of stroke—due to idiopathic primary detrusor instability, prostatic enlargement, oestrogen deficiency, stones, or bladder cancer.
- Incomplete bladder emptying is most often due to prostate disease, faecal impaction, or anticholinergic drugs, but a proportion have idiopathic detrusor underactivity, including some women.
- Dementia is associated with lack of awareness, communication difficulties, bladder instability, disorientation, and agnosia.

Management

- Perform urinalysis, and if abnormal send urine for culture. If there is haematuria this may require investigation. If there is infection, treat it.
- Measure the postvoid residual volume, by ultrasound scan.
- Ensure a reasonable fluid intake—aim for 2L a day plus what comes in food, and avoid caffeine (concentrated urine and caffeine irritate the bladder). However, caffeine withdrawal symptoms can be unpleasant (headache, irritability, poor concentration).
- If possible complete a 3-day frequency–volume chart. This will give an idea of functional bladder capacity (low, often <200mL, in instability), total urine output, and the day–night split of output. If the patient is incontinent into pads, these can be weighed to estimate voided volume.
- If the patient is aphasic, has other communication problems, or dementia, offer the toilet every 2h (they may have bladder instability as well).
- Add an anticholinergic drug if the residual volume is <100mL. The newer bladder-selective drugs provide the best balance between efficacy and side effects (mainly dry mouth and heartburn). Tolterodine XL 4mg od, or trospium 20mg bd are examples. But none of these drugs is dramatically effective. In trials, cystometric bladder capacity

increased from about 200mL to 250mL (normal capacity 400–600mL, a little lower in an older person).

- Vaginal oestrogens sometimes relieve urgency and can be a helpful adjunct (creams are messy—use Vagifem® vaginal tablets).
- Consider the possibility of genuine stress incontinence (leakage on raising abdominal pressure without detrusor contraction). The first-line treatment is pelvic floor re-education. Pelvic floor contraction helps inhibit unstable detrusor contractions, so there is some benefit from pelvic floor exercises regardless of diagnosis. There may be an associated cystocoele which needs diagnosing and appropriate management.
- If there is retention, try a Queens Square Bladder Stimulator (a vibrating massaging device), intermittent catheterization, or an alpha blocker (doxazosin 1mg increasing to 4mg od—needs titrating to avoid postural hypotension, but can be coindicated as antihypertensives, or tamsulosin MR 400mcg od, which is uroselective and has less effect on BP).
- If unsuccessful, optimize containment:
  - For men try a sheath catheter (penile size should not matter).
  - Otherwise try pads. These have a capacity up to 1100ml , but if saturated are heavy (1100g).
  - Indwelling catheters are a last resort. They always get infected, block, or bypass due to bladder spasm. An anticholinergic may be needed for this. Do not shrink from a 'trial of catheter' if that is what the duly-informed patient wants, and it is the only way to get someone home. The usually well-justified reluctance to use catheters can be taken too far.
  - Consider a suprapubic catheter if intended as long term—they are more comfortable and less prone to infection.

Other urinary symptoms can be equally troublesome, in particular urgency and nocturia. The need for multiple transfers onto the commode or trips to the toilet at night is a major falls risk and can place considerable strain on a spouse or cohabiting carer:
- Make continence as easy as possible—use regular prompted voiding, or provide urinals.
- Urgency almost always means detrusor instability, but can sometime indicate incomplete bladder emptying. Do a bladder scan and then give an anticholinergic drug.
- Nocturia can indicate:
  - Unstable bladder—should be detectable from frequent low volume voids on the frequency–volume chart.
  - Nocturnal polyuria—night time (8h whilst asleep) output should be <1/3 of total output. Normal urine output rate is 70–100mL/h— depending on fluid intake. The normal young adult circadian rhythm in ADH-vasopressin secretion reduces this to 35mL/h during sleep. Causes of nocturnal polyuria include diabetes, alcohol consumption, oedema, lithium therapy, heart failure, hypercalcaemia, and, most commonly, age-related nocturnal polyuria. If the latter, this is a combined loss of diurnal variation in vasopressin secretion and partial renal unresponsiveness to it (i.e. partial cranial and partial nephrogenic diabetes insipidus). Try giving chlorthalidone 100mg

bd, decreasing to 50mg od after a month (this has a paradoxical antidiuretic action by sensitizing renal tubules to ADH). It often cuts night-time output by about a half. Furosemide 40mg in the morning sometimes helps, but causes urinary problems of its own. Desmopressin 200–400mcg po given 6 nights in 7 sometimes works, but is often disappointing in practice. Moreover, in the UK it is not licensed for use in people >65 years, who are more prone to hyponatraemia, and who are often hypertensive.

• Insomnia—ask about pain, anxiety, depression.
• Incomplete bladder emptying—will need relieving, medically (alpha blockers), surgically (transurethral resection of the prostate, TURP) or with a catheter (intermittent if possible).

Faecal incontinence

• This is very common in the early period after severe stroke.
• In the longer term, persisting and uncontrolled faecal incontinence is a major barrier to discharge home.
• Seek a cause—(Box 8.6); but don't expect this to be easy.
• Many patients are constipated. The rectum is a mucus-producing organ, and a hard faecal mass stimulates its production, which then leaks out as 'spurious diarrhoea'. A rectal examination, and often an abdominal X-ray are required. Treatment is with laxatives (senna 15–30mg/day, sodium docusate 200mg bd), or enemas. Avoid constipating drugs, and ensure adequate fluid intake. Later on, encourage mobility and adequate dietary fibre.
• A disinhibited colon may recover with time. Apart from excluding constipation, there is nothing to be done in the acute phase. Later on try to anticipate bowel opening (keep a bowel chart). If a discharge depends on continence, initiate a bowel regimen (loperamide 2–16mg/day) to induce constipation, then arrange enemas 2–3 times a week for a controlled bowel evacuation. Patients often find this unpleasant. Otherwise, ensure adequate containment (pads), and that they are changed quickly if soiled.
• Be aware of drug-induced diarrhoea (laxatives, iron, proton pump inhibitors, and metformin).

Box 8.6 Causes of faecal incontinence

- Constipation with overflow incontinence.
- Disinhibited 'neurogenic' colon.
- Diarrhoea.
- Laxatives or other drugs.
- Diminished level of consciousness or unawareness.
- Immobility.

Mood

- 1–4 months after a stroke 10–20% of survivors are depressed and a quarter anxious. Half will recover within a year.
- Depression is strongly associated with physical disability and somatic illness. It is most likely due to loss of abilities, and threats to life, future independence, and ambitions, than anything more 'neurological'.
- Emotional lability, usually inappropriate crying (sometimes anger or laughter), in the absence of a sufficiently strong stimulus, is not the same as depression, but responds well (and quickly) to both SSRIs and tricyclic antidepressants. It affects about 15%, and is often triggered by emotionally-laden questions. The crying is distressing despite its inappropriateness.
- Assessing depression in these circumstances is difficult. Features include persistent:
  - Sadness.
  - Pessimism or hopelessness.
  - Lack of responsiveness to pleasant activities.
  - Inability to concentrate.
  - Irritability.
  - Insomnia.
  - Worry about the future.
- Somatic features like fatigue, sleep disturbance, poor appetite, weight loss, and constipation are too non-specific to be useful in isolation. Inability to enjoy things or undertake previous activities is as likely due to the physical effects of stroke as a mood disorder.
- Aphasia may make assessment almost impossible.
- Depression will often present as a possible explanation for a problem such as lack of motivation, or failure to make progress anticipated.
- Sometimes the diagnosis will be an 'adjustment reaction' (the under-standable psychological response to unpleasant circumstances). This fluctuates day to day, and is distractible.
- Major affective disorder is hard to diagnose in any severe physical illness (Box 8.7). Worthlessness, hopelessness, guilt, and anhedonia are useful pointers, along with the persistence and severity of the symptoms. To make a diagnosis of depression symptoms must persist for at least 2 weeks.
- Therapy is largely unevaluated. All the things that comprise good multidisciplinary care should help (a positive and purposeful approach, identifying and tackling practical problems, and time to talk).
- More structured psychological approaches may help (Box 8.8). 'Problem solving therapy' and 'motivational interviewing' have some evidence for effectiveness.
- Often we resort to a therapeutic trial of antidepressant drugs. But remember these drugs have side effects. SSRIs are the current favour-ites, but their advantages over tricyclics are overstated, and their efficacy is not great. They are at least as likely to cause falls as tricyclics, and various other problems can be seen, including nausea, anxiety, hyponatraemia, delirium, and extrapyramidal movement disorders.

There is little to choose between types. Citalopram (20mg od) is a reasonable choice, and cheap.

- Lofepramine (start at 70mg od, increase up to 210mg/day in split doses), trazodone (50–200mg at night), and dothiepin (50–150mg at night) can be also useful, the last two where anxiety or agitation are problematic, but have anticholinergic side effects and are more cardio-toxic than SSRIs.
- Make sure drugs are stopped if they are ineffective, but give them a decent trial (3 weeks) after titrating up to full dose.

Box 8.7 Diagnostic criteria for major affective disorder

- Usually:
  - Depressed mood—varying little from day to day, or with circum-stances, but often worse in the morning.
  - Loss of interest and enjoyment, loss of response to enjoyable activities, events, or surroundings.
  - Reduced energy, increased fatigability after minimal effort, dimin-ished activity.
- Commonly:
  - Reduced concentration and attention.
  - Reduced self-esteem and self-confidence.
  - Ideas of guilt and worthlessness.
  - Bleak and pessimistic view of the future.
  - Ideas or acts of suicide or self-harm.
  - Disturbed sleep (early morning waking by >2h from usual).
  - Diminished appetite, weight loss of >5% in a month.
  - Loss of libido.
- Atypical features:
  - Anxiety, agitation.
  - Hypersolomnence.
  - Psychomotor retardation.
- Lasting >2 weeks.

ICD-10 Classification of Mental and Behavioural Disorders, WHO, 1992.

Box 8.8 Structured programme to treat poststroke depression

- 188 survivors of ischaemic stroke, who were able to communicate, were not cognitively impaired, and who screened positive for depression on a brief screening tool (9-item Patient Health Questionnaire Depression Scale), were randomized between a care management programme called 'Activate–Initiate–Monitor' (AIM) or usual care. Mean age was 60, 75% had diagnosable DSM-IV major depression, but depression severity was only moderate, and stroke severity was mild (mean NIHSS 3).
- The AIM intervention was conducted by medically-supervised nurse care managers with 3 steps:
  - Activating stroke survivors and their families to understand and accept depression diagnosis and treatment, in a 20-min structured psychoeducational session. The session included discussion of depression diagnosis, symptoms, and treatment guidelines with emphasis on destigmatizing the diagnosis and reinforcing the link between symptoms and treatment.
  - Initiating antidepressant medication; recommendations followed an algorithm, which took into account previous therapy failures, adverse effects or contraindications, but which usually involved initial treatment with an SSRI (usually paroxetine).
  - Monitoring treatment effectiveness by bimonthly telephone calls from the nurse to assess symptoms, side effects, and adherence. Antidepressant dose was increased after 4 weeks of treatment if symptoms were not improving, or changed to an SNRI (usually venlafaxine).
- Usual care included an attention placebo, and antidepressant prescription at the discretion of patient's doctor. In practice, 56% of usual care patients received an antidepressant drug.
- Primary outcome measure was depression response after 12 weeks (Hamilton Depression Inventory score <8 or a decrease from baseline of at least 50%).
- Response was greater in the AIM care management group than usual care:
  - Overall response 51% vs. 30% (P <0.005).
  - Remission (Hamilton score <8): 39% vs. 23% (P <0.01).
- Response was evident by 6 weeks. Adverse effects were no different between groups. 16% of AIM group participants required a change in medication.
- Antidepressant medication should be supported by education, and active follow-up to monitor symptoms, drug effects and side effects, and adjust treatment if necessary.

Stroke 2007; **38**:998–1003.

Communication

(See also 📖 Aphasia, p.73 and p.310).

Aphasia and dysarthria affect 20% of stroke survivors each. Half of people with aphasia will still be aphasic 6 months after a stroke, although dysarthria tends to recover.

Assess both understanding and expression. Be aware of other problems that might complicate an assessment of language function—deafness, concentration, visual problems, cognitive impairment, depression.

Simple tests:
• Assess spontaneous speech.
• Screen for comprehension problems with a complex command (touch your right ear with your left hand).
• Follow-up with simple motor commands (close eyes, show tongue), or 2- and 3-stage commands.
• Questions with yes/no answers.
• Automatic sequences (counting, days of the week).
• Object naming, increasingly difficult (e.g. watch, strap, buckle, winder, hands).
• Repetition.
• Describing a picture.
• Reading and writing.

Discuss functional communication (ability to make needs known, or to follow or cooperate with requests) with other team members.

Speech and language therapists will give a detailed and systematic assessment of the language problem, which can be useful in helping the rest of the team (and relatives) understand the problem. They can also advise on communication aids (e.g. picture boards), pacing of speech, and non-verbal cues. All staff should have a basic understanding of these.

At least as valuable a function as improving language is the provision of explanation and support. Language disorders are generally not well understood, and may be mistaken for dementia. Severe aphasia is immensely frustrating for both patient and carers. Emotional support, practical advice, and contact with other people with similar problems are all required.

How to talk to someone with aphasia—see 📖 Aphasia, p.73.

Activities of daily living

Occupational therapists and nurses are the key, but teamwork remains important. Dressing is hard if the patient cannot stand up, or is dizzy or breathless.

The approach to solving problems is:
- To identify the activity (or level of activity) required or desired, and set goals.
- Recognize the problems in achieving it, and anticipate how these problems (e.g. limb weakness) may change.
- Identify any aids or adaptations necessary to make the task easier or safer.
- Teach new ways of doing the task. This may involve breaking a task down into smaller steps, practising sequencing, and techniques like verbalizing if dyspraxic.
- Practise it.
- Identify barriers that other disciplines may help overcome (e.g. nocturia due to polyuria or unstable bladder, standing difficulties due to heel sores), and liaise with the appropriate person.
- Assess how the function will be undertaken in the home environment, including work with family, other professionals, or carers (training in transfers, including using a rotunda or hoist, managing stoma or catheter bags, advice on food and fluids consistencies and safe swallowing tips, or delivering PEG feeds).

These may be backed up by home visiting, or in rehabilitation follow-up.

Falls and fractures

- Falls and fractures are a particular concern after strokes.
- Osteoporosis is common amongst the older (especially female) population, and is worse in hemiparetic limbs.
  - Over half this population will have biochemical vitamin D deficiency, or insufficiency (suboptimal vitamin D levels from the point of view of bone health, with secondary hyperparathyroidism, but not overt deficiency). Many stroke patients benefit from vitamin D supplementation, such as a combined high-dose calcium (1g/day) and vitamin D tablet (800IU/day).
- Patients with a history of low trauma fracture or kyphosis are candidates for a bisphosphonate (alendronate 70mg weekly). Alternatives include IV ibandronate (3mg given 3-monthly), IV zolendronic acid (5mg given yearly), raloxifene (60mg od), or strontium ranelate (2g od).
- Multifactorial falls prevention should be undertaken:
  - Diagnose postural dizziness or syncope.
  - Check for postural hypotension.
  - Medication review avoiding neuroleptics, sedatives, antidepressants (and hypotensive drugs in the presence of postural hypotension).
  - Advise getting up from bed or chair slowly.
  - Check for cataracts.
  - Up-to-date glasses.
  - Optimize gait pattern and transfer technique.
  - Muscle strength and balance training.
  - Check for foot problems and arrange chiropody.
  - Diagnose and treat nocturia.
  - Optimize lighting.
  - Minimize environmental hazards.
- Remember that the immediate risk from a fall due to postural hypotension (1–2% risk of hip fracture, 5% risk of other fracture, 10% chance serious injury per fall) is greater than the future risk of stroke from hypertension.
- A patient who is falling frequently may like to try mechanical hip protectors (pants with plastic 'shin-pads' sewn in over the greater trochanters). For those who actually wear them regularly (many find them too uncomfortable), these may provide protection against hip fracture. But they are expensive (£40 a pair), and you need three pairs (one on, one in the wash, one for tomorrow).

Body image

Facial droop, speech problems, abnormal posture or gait attract stigma. Able-bodied people tend to 'talk over' people with disabilities rather than talking to them, and may avoid them altogether. Professional staff must try not to fall into the same trap. Psychological readjustment requires restoring self-confidence and esteem:

- Encourage wearing of own clothes, taking pride in appearance, and using make-up if preferred.
- Talk to patients as sensible adults.
- Make compliments and positive comments.
- Encourage family and visitors to do the same, and point it out if they do not.
- Communal meals can help.
- Offer tissues for drooling.
- Encourage use of glasses or hearing aid.
- Make sure nails are cut, and shaving done properly.
- Ensure the privacy that is usually expected for washing and going to the toilet. Avoid commodes if possible.
- Ensure the availability of appropriate feeding aids, change clothes after food spills.
- Respect cultural needs and differences.

Family and carer involvement in rehabilitation

Family involvement, with an emphasis on information and education, is a key feature of successful stroke units (Box 8.9). This should include:

- Information on stroke and its consequences, prevention, and management options.
- Involvement in goal setting for rehabilitation and discharge planning.
- Encouragement to attend nursing and therapy activities to learn about patients' abilities, and instruction on managing transfers, mobility, and ADL.
- Prewarning about potential sources of stress and coping strategies.
- Advice on community services, benefits, allowances, and voluntary support services for carers.

This serves to support and encourage the patient emotionally, increase confidence in family and carers, individualize rehabilitation goals, identify unexpected problems, prepare carers for tasks that they may need to undertake at home (remembering that spouses may be elderly and in poor health themselves), increase a sense of responsibility and control, and reduce over protectiveness.

Information and education interventions should be targeted and interactive (directed at specific problems faced by the patient, and actively engaging the patient or carer) rather than simply issuing leaflets (although written information is also valuable).

Box 8.9 Training carers of stroke patients

- 300 stroke patients and their informal carers (two-thirds of whom were spouses) were randomized between conventional care and participation in an additional training programme.
- Patients were treated on a stroke unit, and had residual disability (requiring supervision or assistance in basic ADL), but were expected to be discharged home.
- Normal stroke unit care included extensive family and carer involvement, including informal involvement in therapy and nursing care, and advice on community services.
- The additional training included:
  - Instruction by therapists or nurses on common stroke-related problems and their prevention, risk of pressure sores, continence, nutrition, positioning, how to help with walking, and advice on benefits and local services.
  - 'Hands-on' training in lifting and handling, mobility and transfers, continence, assistance with personal ADL and communication, tailored to the needs of individual patients.
  - Training started when patients' rehabilitation needs had stabilized and discharge was contemplated. Carers received three to five sessions depending on need. Each session lasted 30–45min. Carers' competencies were assessed at the end of training. In addition the hospital team conducted a follow-up session at home to adapt skills learnt to the home environment.
- Outcomes were measured at 3 and 12 months:
  - Trained carers experienced less carer burden (score 32 vs 41; p=0.0001), anxiety (score 3 vs 4; p=0.0001), or depression (score 2 vs 3; p=0.0001) and had a higher quality of life (EuroQol visual analogue scale score 80 vs 70; p=0.001).
  - Patients reported less anxiety (3 vs 4.5; p <0.0001) and depression (3 vs 4; p <0.0001) and better quality of life (Euroqol 65 vs 60; p=0.009) in the caregiver training group.
  - Patients' mortality, institutionalization, and disability were not influenced by caregiver training.
- Costs of care over 1 year for patients whose carers had received training were lower.

British Medical Journal 2004; **328**:1099–104.

Where to do rehabilitation

Inpatient hospital wards

Conventionally, rehabilitation has taken place on specialist hospital wards (stroke units or mixed rehabilitation wards). There is good evidence that these improve outcomes—about a 20–30% reduction in risk of death, dependency, or institutional care compared with 'standard care' on a general medical ward (see 📖 Box 3.3, p.92).

Some models have mixed acute and rehabilitation stroke wards, acknowledging that the transition from 'acute' to 'rehabilitation' is arbitrary. On the other hand, some aspects of acute care (intensive monitoring, dealing with parenteral infusions) can detract from rehabilitation nursing. So other models separate these functions, whilst recognizing that staff dealing with acute stroke should be trained in rehabilitation, and adequate therapy provision is made on acute wards to cover this function.

Inpatient stroke unit rehabilitation is the current 'gold standard of care' against which innovations must be compared.

Home rehabilitation

If a patient is able to transfer alone, or with the help of a willing carer (to allow them to get to the toilet in the night), and has sufficient insight and judgement to maintain safety if left alone for a few hours, then home rehabilitation is feasible if there is a service locally. This care divides between 'early discharge' schemes designed to expedite hospital discharge, and longer-term community support and rehabilitation services (see 📖 Box 9.1, p.221).

Home therapy has potential advantages—such as working on activities in the environment in which they will eventually have to be performed, with the people and resources likely to be available to help, as well as avoiding the unpleasantness of hospital wards and ambulance journeys.

Other forms of 'intermediate care'

In the UK these are defined as short-term rehabilitation schemes, designed to prevent hospital admission, expedite hospital discharge, or provide postdischarge rehabilitation after an episode of acute illness. Such care may be provided in residential or nursing homes, and may also include the types of home rehabilitation described earlier. From the point of view of stroke, the short time-frame limits applicability for the most affected patients, but may provide a useful stepping stone on the way home for some.

Anticipating longer-term problems

Patients and carers often report being underprepared for the return home, and the problems to be faced in the longer term. Teaching and training can help (see 📖 p.215).

Hospital staff can help if they too know what to expect. Close liaison with early discharge and community rehabilitation teams, and voluntary sector support organizations, can provide educational opportunities. Some of the issues are discussed in 📖 Chapter 12, pp.297–322.

Summary

1. Rehabilitation is the process of restoring functional ability after an illness, and then helping the patient to come to terms with ongoing disability.
2. Interventions include preventing or treating pathologies (or complications), relieving impairments, and remediating disabilities, taking full account of the social and physical environment.
3. It is necessarily multidisciplinary, and members should work together as a team, communicating regularly and systematically.
4. Problems should be identified and goals set, in order to evaluate progress and identify complications or setbacks.
5. Rehabilitation should occur in the place most appropriate to the particular problems identified, including at home.
5. Mobility, continence, psychological and behavioural problems are central to successful rehabilitation, and require expert assessment and management.
6. Specific programmes of patient and carer education and training reduces carer strain and improves later psychological health
7. Psychological adjustment is central to longer-term well-being, but is usually addressed patchily, if at all. In hospital, measures to promote positive body image and self-esteem, and attempts to anticipate later problems, facilitate the adjustment process.

Chapter 9

Discharge

When is it time for discharge?

The time for hospital discharge is when what is needed can be provided elsewhere.

If you are going to stay in hospital it has to be for a purpose—mainly because hospitals are no place to live a life, but also because beds represent a scare resource. Reasons for being in hospital include:

- Nursing care (feeding, washing, hygiene, basic mobility, protecting pressures areas, avoidance of other complications, delivering medication), especially where care is required unpredictably or intensively 24h a day.
- Access to diagnostic tests, not available outside hospital.
- Access to medical treatments (of stroke or complications), not available outside hospital.
- Delivery of rehabilitation.
- Waiting—for tests, treatment, or for home or institutional care to be organized or available.
- Convenience of not requiring multiple trips to hospital for tests or therapy or medical consultations.

Much nursing and rehabilitation can be delivered at home. Increasingly, community services are available which can do this (Box 9.1). This is not an excuse for indiscriminate off-loading of patients. The gold-standard for acute and rehabilitation care is an inpatient stroke unit. Any community rehabilitation scheme must match (or exceed) what a stroke unit can provide. This means:

- Multidisciplinary staffing, with occupational therapy, physiotherapy, nursing, speech and language therapy, and access to dietetics, social work, clinical psychology, or mental health nursing, if needed.
- Consultant medical support.
- Therapy support workers, either discipline-specific or, more usually, generic rehabilitation assistants.
- Adequate numbers of staff to provide as much therapy as the patient can tolerate.
- Multidisciplinary meetings to communicate, coordinate, identify problems, set goals, monitor progress, and plan eventual discharge.

Box 9.1 South London Early Discharge Scheme for stroke

- 331 patients (about half the stroke admissions during the study) were allocated to home rehabilitation for 3 months, or to further hospital care. The criterion for inclusion was ability to transfer from bed to chair independently or with the help of a willing carer. Half the hospital care group were treated on a stroke unit.
- Home care was individualized, with up to one visit per day from each of physiotherapy and occupational therapy, plus up to 3h daily of Social Services generic personal care.
- 1 year later, there were no differences in outcomes (motor weakness, 5-metre timed walk, disability (Barthel Index), cognition, anxiety and depression, carer strain, and satisfaction).
- On average, 6 days' hospital stay per patient randomized were saved.

British Medical Journal 1997, **315**.1039–44.

Is discharge safe?

Consider fitness for discharge at the levels of:
- The person.
- Their abilities.
- The environment.

At the person level, this will mean being 'medically stable':
- In a stable cardiac rhythm, with adequate BP, free from severe heart failure or any life-threatening cardiovascular problems (acute coronary syndrome, tamponade).
- Adequate, and stable, respiratory function.
- Free from acute renal failure, or other severe metabolic derangement such as severe dehydration, electrolyte or glucose disturbance.
- Free from severe infection.
- Able to swallow safely, or having a means of non-oral feeding (i.e. a PEG tube).
- Free from severe debilitating symptoms such as frequent fits, pain, nausea, or breathlessness.

At the level of activities, at a minimum, it will require:
- Ability to transfer from bed to chair, wheelchair or commode, alone or with a willing and able carer (with a hoist if necessary).
- Continence, or adequate containment.
- Measures to relieve skin pressure.
- Ability, judgement, and insight to avoid falls, injury, or other safety problems.
- Ability to take prescribed drugs, or someone to supervise them.

The environment divides into the physical and social environment:
- Sufficient human help—full-time, if help may be required urgently or unpredictably; otherwise sufficient to ensure:
  - Toileting.
  - Pressure area care.
  - Feeding and hygiene.
  - Occupation.
  - Social and emotional contact.
- Adequate equipment, including:
  - Suitable bed and chair.
  - Pressure-relieving mattress and cushions.
  - Commode, urinals, or bedpan.
  - Feeding equipment (e.g. feeding pumps for PEG feeds).
  - Pendant alarm or mobile phone if left alone for periods of time.
  - Means of entry for care staff if living alone (key safe or door entry system).
  - Mobility aids (wheelchair, sticks, frame; rotunda, sliding board or hoist for transfers).
  - Rails to facilitate bed and toilet transfers.

Exceptions:
- In some cases, such as discharge for home terminal care, safety (in terms of protecting life) is not a prime concern. But many of the same considerations are needed to make the discharge practical and humane.

- Hospital is not a prison. Patients cannot be detained unless they consent, or have been shown to lack capacity and remaining in hospital is in their best interests. Remember that capacity must be assumed unless it can be demonstrated otherwise.
- Health and Safety legislation applies to professional and home care staff. They cannot therefore undertake tasks carrying undue risk—for example, manual transfers represent a risk of back injury, and a hoist may be required. If the patient refuses a hoist, or there is no room, in, for example, a cramped bedroom, and alternative arrangements cannot be made, staff cannot be expected to undertake transfers. Other sources of risk include aggressive or disinhibited patients with cognitive impairment.

Is appropriate community support and follow-up available?

If there are unmet rehabilitation needs, and these cannot be provided outside of hospital, then offer to provide them in hospital. Otherwise community support divides into therapeutic services (trying to improve function), and prosthetic services (making up for things the person cannot do themselves).

Therapeutic services include:
- Early discharge support and rehabilitation teams.
- Longer-term stroke disability support and rehabilitation services.
- Day hospitals.
- Generic community services such as family doctors, district nursing, community physiotherapy, Social Services occupational therapy (who are responsible for providing many aids and home adaptations), and speech and language therapy.
- 'Intermediate care', based in residential or nursing homes. Care must be taken to ensure that these are genuinely specialist stroke rehabilitation services, not just a convenient way of freeing up hospital beds. These services will often have scant medical and nursing staffing, and may need to be considered the equivalent of 'home' discharges.

Prosthetic services include:
- Social Services home care, including help to get up and be put to bed, washing and dressing, get meals, empty catheter bags or commodes, supervise medication, housework, and shopping.
- Meals at home service (from Social Services, or private equivalents, or someone to buy 'ready meals' at the supermarket and a microwave to heat them in).
- Day centres.
- Visitor and advocate schemes.
- Sitting services for carers.
- Respite care in residential or nursing homes.
- Permanent placement in a residential or nursing home.

Are the carers prepared?

The presence of a willing carer can enable a discharge which would otherwise be impossible. Such carers:

- Provide hands-on care, in much the same way as Social Services home care—transferring, toileting, catheter care and changing pads, getting meals, other domestic tasks, operating feeding pumps for PEG tubes, giving medication.
- Providing supervision and surveillance, looking out for problems.
- Providing company, occupation, and emotional support.

The commitment of some carers, and the range of tasks they will take on, is sometimes staggering. Many of these are tasks that previous everyday life has not prepared them for, such as:

- Catheter and PEG tube care.
- Safe transfers (safe for both patient and carer), or operating a hoist.
- Supervised walking.
- Dressing, and the tricks required to dress a hemiplegic person successfully (paralysed side on first and off last).
- Feeding, sometimes in patients with precarious swallowing, who need advice on positioning, consistencies, and pacing of feeds.
- Pressure area care, including turning, and operating pressure-relieving mattresses.
- Administration of medicines, including insulin.
- Intermittent urinary catheterization.

These needs should be anticipated during rehabilitation, and carers given appropriate training, by occupational therapy, physiotherapy, and nursing staff (see 📖 Chapter 8, p.177 and Box 8.9, p.215).

Elderly spouses are sometimes frail themselves. Statutory services may be required to support an 'informal' carer:

- In the UK, carers have a statutory right to have their own needs assessed by Social Services departments.
- Respite care (a period in a residential or nursing home, or sometimes a hospital, to give carers a holiday or break) may need to be anticipated and arranged.
- Sitting services can allow a carer a few hours to go shopping, or to pursue social or leisure activities of their own. Opportunities for these can become very limited when caring for a very dependent person.

Is the environment optimized?

Environments can facilitate activity and participation, or provide a barrier to it. Examples include access ramps, stair rails or stair lifts, grab rails around toilets and baths, bathing equipment such as bath boards, 'glide about' chairs (with wheels on) for use in a shower, or 'bed leavers' (a rail by the bed supported under the mattress).

Wheelchair users will need sufficient space to manoeuvre, doors which are wide enough to get through, and toilets with enough space to allow safe transfers. Kitchen work surfaces may need to be lower to allow use.

Home visits by occupational therapists, with or without the patient, a physiotherapist, members of the patient's family, and representatives of Social Services are immensely useful, and serve several purposes:
• An assessment of the physical environment, to look for hazards and other barriers.
• To plan therapeutic changes to the environment (ramps and rails, replacing or altering beds and chairs, recommending improved lighting, removal of clutter, loose wires, and rugs, acquiring kitchen aids).
• Assessing the patient's performance of tasks in the home environment.
• Assessing the viability of community rehabilitation.
• To motivate and encourage the patient, as a clear indication that progress is being made, and discharge planning is taking place.
• To boost the confidence of patient and family or other carers, not least to show that proper planning is taking place.
• To demonstrate that someone will not manage at home, especially if there is dispute about this (whilst realizing safety is a relative and graded phenomenon, not absolute, and that a single home visit will never give a definitive assessment).

Alternative assessment opportunities include:
• Trial periods in a 'rehabilitation flat' attached to a rehabilitation unit. This can be alone, or with a carer such as a spouse. Routine professional input is limited to what a home-care package might provide.
• Overnight stay at home.
• 'Weekend leave' (i.e. several nights, sometimes as part of a 'staged discharge').

These can be used to provide information (will it work?) and to boost confidence.

Institutional discharge

The ultimate in 'environmental modification' is to abandon the previous home environment altogether, and discharge to a residential or nursing home. As a general rule, rehabilitation tries hard to avoid (or defer) this.

Residential homes were originally modelled (in the 1940s) on seaside hotels (to which elderly people would retire). The current definition is that they provide 'board, lodging, and personal care'. However, typically the prevalence of incontinence, dementia, and impaired mobility in these homes is about a third each, indicating substantial nursing and medical needs. Many residents will have developed these conditions since being admitted.

Nursing homes have at least one qualified nurse on duty all the time.

Many homes are 'dual registered' as both residential and nursing homes, and in the UK the distinction between the two is fast becoming blurred, a process largely driven by local authority payers keen to reduce costs.

With sufficient resources, it should theoretically be possible to discharge anyone home. Often institutional discharge is required when disabilities are such that adequate care cannot be provided at home within the budget available. Dementia leading to lack of judgement and safety awareness is often the deciding factor. Onset of faecal incontinence is another particular problem at home. Sometimes people decide that living at home is too dangerous or lonely. Confidence may be lost, especially if a trial of discharge ends in a fall or inability to cope. Where health has been failing for some time before the stroke, institutional care may have been contemplated prior to the stroke. Sometimes relatives push hard for institutional discharge. They will often be influential with patients, but ultimately a patient with capacity has to decide for themselves what they want, and staff should support them in this.

Sometimes people become dead-set on entry to a residential home, when the assessment of professional staff is that they could be managed at home. If the patient is paying for the care themselves, there is nothing to stop them living where they want to. But for people without means, whose care would be funded by Social Services departments, they would be assessed against eligibility criteria, and those assessed as suitable for home care may not be funded.

There can be a major problem in finding somewhere for a severely disabled younger person to live. If home discharge is impossible, there are a few nursing and residential homes specializing in the care of younger people, NHS younger disabled units, and some charities (like the Cheshire Homes) may help.

Is there a need for follow-up?

Follow-up may be:
- Medical, to check on risk factors and secondary prevention, to fol-low-up the results of tests, or to check residual disability or mood.
- One of the therapies, for ongoing rehabilitation needs. A 'need' for healthcare implies the capacity to benefit from an intervention. This implies that someone has ongoing problems, has not reached a 'plateau', and wants to continue therapy. This may be provided in a day hospital, outpatient, or home setting.
- Supportive—such as that provided by aphasia support groups.
- To reassess for ongoing or new disabilities, problems, or mood disorders.
- Generic—patients will continue to have access to primary healthcare teams, who may refer back to specialist services if required.

Capacity and consent

Sometimes people insist on going home when rehabilitation staff are sure that they will not cope. This is usually in the context of dementia, but may occur in anosognosia (denial of stroke) and some other mental illnesses:

- If the patient has mental capacity to give or withhold consent, there is no question. You make things as safe as possible, in terms of environmental modification and prosthetic care, and do as the patient asks.
- If capacity is lacking, you must act in the patient's best interest. Assessing capacity and best interest in these situations can be difficult. We should assume that a patient *has* capacity, *unless* we can show that they do not. The least restrictive approach is to allow the patient to try at home—once at least.
- A second opinion (usually from a psychiatrist) is a sensible safeguard of the patient's rights (you are either considering detaining them against their will, or letting themselves be exposed to undue risk of injury).
- The views of relatives should be sought, especially as they may be required to provide a lot of the ongoing care. They may be as exasperated and helpless as you are. People with dementia are not often amenable to reasoned arguments, although some can be persuaded to have a 'trial' in a residential home. Economy with the truth is a necessary evil here—usually these are people who have settled well into the institutional hospital environment, and would likely be equally happy in a residential home. In the UK, those without family must be referred to an Independent Mental Capacity Advocate.
- If a trial at home fails, and the patient is still insistent that they want to go home, you can argue that they have demonstrated sufficient lack of insight and judgement to show that they do not appreciate the consequences of their request, and therefore lack capacity. These cases can be come quite intractable. You may agree to another trial at home, especially if the circumstances of the previous failure are unlikely to recur.
- There will come a stage, however, sometimes even without a first trial at home, where it is simply irresponsible to allow some one to put themselves in a position of physical danger (falling, wandering, kettles, gas, and fires), and you have to say 'no'. In the UK, this may be the subject of Deprivation of Liberty safeguard procedures.
- The law on consent in this area is very vague. 'Persuasion' and not a little subterfuge are the mainstays of engineering what most objective observers would agree is a sensible solution. These matters cannot be taken lightly in a free country.
- We are unaware of anyone ever having been sued for irresponsibly discharging a patient who has requested it. The Courts are very supportive of professional staff acting reasonably in good faith.

Communicating with primary care—discharge summaries

Hospital doctors should communicate the details of an episode of hospital care to GPs. This also forms the definitive hospital record of the episode.

If a discharge is particularly difficult or contentious, telephone the GP in advance:
- To warn them in case something goes wrong quickly.
- They may want to visit the patient, especially if he or she is dying.
- If you want them to do something.

To be really useful a discharge summary should:
- Be typed, and confined to one side of A4 paper.
- Should reach the GP within a week of discharge (that's what GPs say they need).
- Arrive electronically, to allow uploading to their computer systems.
- Include details of the date of admissions and discharge, which wards were used, and which consultants were responsible.
- The diagnosis responsible for the current admission (but remember not all GPs will know all the fashionable hospital abbreviations, so spell them out).
- All other active or relevant previous diagnoses.
- A description of the problem leading to admission, a brief history of the problem, relevant risk factors, relevant previous functional and social circumstances.
- Relevant physical signs. Include sufficient neurological details to substantiate the OCSP stroke syndrome diagnosed, a MMSE score if done, and details of the ward BP record (a better indication of 'usual' BP than most one-off, 'casual', BP readings).
- Important investigations. Summarize (e.g. 'liver function normal'), but include information relevant to making the diagnosis (CT or MRI result), and secondary prevention (carotid duplex, ECG, echocardiography, cholesterol).
- A summary of treatment and progress, including complications, and failed treatments (intolerance of drugs, measures for restoring continence or controlling pain), functional abilities prior to discharge, and discharge arrangements. If drugs were stopped, say so and why.
- Management plan and follow-up arrangements.
- Drugs on discharge.

Difficulties arise when the 'episode' is incomplete, and follow-up rehabilitation is occurring elsewhere, especially community services and day hospitals, and the hospital notes follow the patient to the new service. In these cases try to do the discharge summary on the day of discharge. Copy the discharge summary to involved health agencies (such as community rehabilitation), and remember that if the patient is discharged to institutional care they may change their GP.

Other primary care agencies (e.g. district nursing) also require handover information where they are to be involved. Information is required on mobility, continence, ADL, wound care and dressings, specific medication problems (such as anticipated compliance problems, or arrangements for drawing-up insulin injections), living arrangements, and other support services involved. GPs often find this information useful as well.

Electronic Patient Records (for hospital), Electronic Health Records (for the whole health system), and unified health and social care records ('Single Assessment Process') may alter the details of how the discharge summary is done, but the information contained will need to be the same.

Summary

1. The time for hospital discharge is when what is needed can be provided elsewhere. Hospital stay has to be well justified.
2. Much nursing and rehabilitation can be delivered at home if (and only if) there are suitable services set up locally.
3. There is no such thing as a safe discharge. There is always a degree of risk. To minimize risk requires that the patient is medically stable, has minimum levels of ability covering mobility, safety awareness, and plans for toileting or containment of incontinence, and necessary equipment, human help, and environmental modifications arranged.
4. Home assessment visits are very useful, but are labour intensive and time consuming.
5. Appropriate follow-up and community support must be arranged. The term 'discharge' is sometimes frowned upon, 'transfer of care' being preferred, as it conveys a suitable concern for continuity. Carers must be prepared.
6. Where capacity to decide is lacking, and the patient wants to try a discharge which is considered high risk, you must assess best interests, but may have to go along with it at least once. Some attempts at discharge are so risky as to be irresponsible.
7. Communicate rapidly and comprehensively with primary healthcare teams.

Chapter 10

Preventing strokes and other vascular events

Vascular risks

- One in five strokes is a recurrent stroke.
- Someone who has had a first stroke is at 10-fold increased risk of another.
- Secondary prevention attempts to reduce the risk of recurrence.
- People with ischaemic heart disease and peripheral vascular disease are more likely to have a stroke, and those who have had a stroke have an increased risk of heart attack. It makes sense to consider vascular prevention all together. The interventions are nearly identical in any case.

The distinction between primary and secondary prevention has been mostly abandoned in recent years. Think of it this way:
- A preventative treatment reduces risk by a certain proportion, on average (1 − relative risk [RR] on treatment).
- How much benefit each individual gets, depends on their chances of having a vascular event at baseline (off treatment):

    Absolute risk reduction = baseline risk × (1 − RR on treatment)

- Baseline risk is determined by previous events, age, sex, and other risk factors such as BP, smoking, and diabetes.

We also know that:
- Most risk factors are not just present or absent, but risk increases with the amount of exposure (BP, cholesterol, number of cigarettes smoked per day, blood glucose, body mass index).
- A lot of risk factors are related to each other (BP is affected by body mass index, diet, alcohol consumption, and physical activity), and some cluster together (diabetics often have raised BP and cholesterol; people who smoke are often overweight).

The effects of risk factors combine together to give an overall risk:
- The Framingham risk equations (📖 Appendices 13 and 14, p.344) put some numbers on the risk (but may overestimate risk in today's population).
- Depending on how much effort and expense (money, inconvenience, side effects) you are willing to commit to prevention (as individuals and as a society), a risk of 15–30% over 10 years is worth intervention. This is not a matter of rationing. 15% risk over 10 years is a *low risk for the individual concerned,* for someone being asked to change lifestyle, or take several drugs a day for all that time.
- If someone has symptomatic vascular disease (diagnosed stroke, ischaemic heart disease, or peripheral vascular disease), their future risk almost invariably puts them in the group where prevention is justified. Most middle-aged or elderly diabetics are as well.
- Risk scores are inevitably crude, and will not include some important risk factors (or diagnoses) which are too rare to have much of an impact on population risk.

Interventions to reduce risk (Table 10.1) divide between:
- General vascular prevention (in common with ischaemic heart disease and peripheral vascular disease):
  - Antithrombotic drugs.
  - BP reduction.
  - Cholesterol reduction.

- Smoking cessation.
- Other lifestyle interventions.
- Stroke-specific interventions:
  - Carotid endarterectomy for severe stenosis.
  - Warfarin in AF.

Table 10.1 Summary of interventions to prevent stroke

Risk factor	Intervention	Evidence	Approximate RR on treatment
Lifestyle factors			
Smoking	Stopping	Cohort studies	0.5 after 2 years
Inactivity	Moderate exercise	Cohort studies	0.5–0.7 in various studies
Salt intake	Reduction	Systematic review of RCTs, BP end-point, single cardiovascular end-point RCT	0.75 per 50mmol Na/day
Obesity	Weight loss	Cohort studies	0.5 per 6kg/m^2
Drug interventions			
BP	Drugs	Systematic reviews of RCTs	0.6 per 10/5mmHg reduction
Isolated systolic hypertension	Drugs	2 RCTs	0.6 for 12mmHg systolic fall
Cholesterol	HMGCoA reductase inhibitors ('statins')	Systematic reviews of RCTs	0.75 (any vascular event)
AF	Warfarin (INR 2–3)	Systematic reviews of RCTs	0.3
AF	Aspirin	Systematic reviews of RCTs	0.8
TIA/ minor stroke	Aspirin/ dipyridamole or clopidogrel	Systematic reviews of RCTs	0.7
Post MI	Warfarin	Systematic reviews of RCTs	0.5

Table 10.1 *(Contd.)*

Risk factor	Intervention	Evidence	Approximate RR on treatment
Surgical interventions			
Symptomatic carotid stenosis (70–99%)	Surgery (vs medical)	Systematic reviews of RCTs	0.5 (after 5 years incl. surgical mortality/ morbidity)*
Asymptomatic carotid stenosis (60–99%)	Surgery (vs medical)	2 RCTs	0.5 (after 5 years incl. surgical mortality/ morbidity)*

*The effect of these interventions cannot be described by a single RR. Surgical morbidity produces an immediate hazard after which strokes accumulate more slowly in surgical patients. HMGCoA, hydroxymethylglutaryl-coenzyme A; RCT, randomized controlled trial.

Box 10.1 Understanding trials in vascular prevention

Why randomized trials?
- Trials aim to establish a causal association between a treatment and an outcome.
- Random allocation aims to ensure that comparison groups are alike in all respects apart from the trial treatment they receive—i.e. the comparison is free from 'bias' and 'confounding'.

The results of a trial
- The main result is the size of the difference in outcomes between the treatments. This can be: the absolute difference in proportions experiencing an outcome (e.g. death, stroke, any cardiovascular event); or the RR of an outcome (also called the risk ratio, rate ratio, odds ratio, or hazard ratio depending on how the calculations were done).
- RR reduction is often quoted. This is (1 − RR), expressed as a percentage. This number usually looks more impressive than the absolute risk difference or the RR!
- The p-value tells you nothing about the size of the treatment effect.
- The numbers needed to treat (NNT) is the number of people who must be given a treatment for 1 year to prevent one event (or cause one adverse effect). It may be quoted over 5 or 10 years, in which case the NNT is 5 or 10 times less.
- NNT is (1/absolute risk difference) given the baseline risk *in the population you are interested in*. This can be estimated as 1/(estimated baseline risk × RR reduction).

Why do trials need to be big?
- Trials must be large enough to be able to measure small differences, e.g. in the Heart Protection Study all-cause mortality was reduced from 14.7% to 12.9%.
- The larger the trial, the less likely that measured differences are of the size that might also have occurred by chance. This is called the power of the trial.

- The power of the trial actually depends on the number of outcome events. A smaller trial of high-risk patients may be more powerful than a large trial of low-risk patients. To maximize power a 'combined vascular end-point' (e.g. fatal and non-fatal heart attack and stroke, vascular deaths, revascularizations and vascular amputations). This is reasonable, but look to see which components are actually showing differences as well.

p-values
- The probability that an observed difference could have arisen by chance is the p-value.
- A non-significant p-value does not mean there is no difference. Look at the 95% CI of the difference between treatment arms or the RR, to see how big or small the real difference could be.
- A significant p-value in a large trial does not tell you whether the size of the effect is of any clinical importance or not.

Intention to treat analysis
- A trial will underestimate the true effect of a treatment ('null bias') because of drop-outs and cross-overs (some placebo-assigned patients will get the treatment outside the trial, some active treatment-assigned patients will stop taking it).
- Trials are analysed according to 'intention to treat' (ITT) not 'treatment received'. This means that a placebo-assigned patient will be analysed as if they did not get the treatment, even if they receive the treatment outside the trial. Treatment-assigned subjects are analysed as if they received treatment, even if they never took it.
- The reason for ITT is to minimize the possibility of bias. People who drop out or cross-over are not representative of the group as a whole. For example, in a BP trial the placebo-assigned patients who are given active treatment outside the trial are likely to be those with the highest BPs, who are also the most likely to have a stroke. You cannot identify the patients in the active treatment group who 'match' these cross-over patients. They remain included in the treatment arm. If you exclude cross-over patients, or worse still, re-assign them to the active treatment arm, you are no longer comparing like with like in terms of initial risk. The final comparison will be biased (in this example, against demonstrating an effect of the active treatment).
- An 'on treatment', or 'per protocol' analysis will often overestimate the effect of the treatment, and is only useful if you are trying to demonstrate it has no effect. In all other cases disregard such results.
- ITT to some extent replicates clinical practice when compliance is uncertain. However, this is not the main reason for doing ITT analyses.

Indirect comparisons of trial results
- The size of effect seen in any one trial will vary by chance. Indirect comparisons of different agents will often be made (especially by drug companies whose drug appears to be better), but these can be misleading.

(Continued)

Box 10.1 *(Contd.)*

- The best way to tell if any one treatment is really different from similar treatments is to look for a statistical test for heterogeneity in a meta-analysis of several treatment trials.
- Head-to-head comparisons of active agents are more reliable, but are fairly rare, since they need to be very large to show differences.

Practical issues

- Comparison of different agents in BP trials is complicated by the need to tailor regimens according to coindications and adverse effects, and use drugs in combination to get adequate response.

Box 10.2 Systematic review and meta-analysis

- Systematic reviews attempt to identify all trial data, published and unpublished, evaluating an intervention. Meta-analysis is a statistical technique for combining data into an overall estimate of effect. Ideally this is done by retrieving individual patient data from investigators, but can also be done from published summary reports.
- The advantage is that with more outcome events, estimates of effect are more powerful (more likely to detect a real difference), and more precise (estimating the size of the effect better). This reduces the effect of random variation in the size of differences seen in trials.
- Meta-regression can use differences between trials (e.g. the population, setting, or precise drug used) to identify which factors influence the overall result.
- The disadvantage is 'heterogeneity'—you may not be comparing like with like when you combine data from two or more trials. This can be tested for statistically. However, lack of heterogeneity can provide evidence (albeit weak) that the interventions in component trials are no different (e.g. different drugs to reduce BP).
- Results are prone to publication bias (negative trials are less likely to be published), and tests (a funnel plot) can be done to assess the likelihood of this.

Antithrombotics

- Aspirin reduces (ischaemic) vascular risk by about 25%. The evidence for giving 75mg of aspirin is as strong as for any other dose (Box10.3).
- 75mg/day of aspirin doubles risk of peptic ulcer disease complications (bleeding, perforation). The incidence of side effects increases rapidly with higher doses.
- Two large trials demonstrated additional benefit for aspirin plus MR dipyridamole over aspirin alone, amongst patients with ischaemic stroke or TIA (Box10.4).
- Clopidogrel is marginally more effective than aspirin, but is very expensive. Use it in cases of true aspirin intolerance (allergy, aspirin-induced asthma, or intractable dyspepsia despite coadministration of a proton pump inhibitor).
- There is no difference in efficacy between aspirin/dipyridamole combination and clopidogrel alone. Adding clopidogrel to aspirin produces no net benefit (or harm) over 18 months of treatment.
- Warfarin (INR 1.4–3), in the absence of AF, reduces infarcts, but the benefit is offset by excess bleeds, and there is no net benefit over antiplatelet therapy (but no harm, either).
- Warfarin (INR 3–4) causes more intracerebral bleeds than it prevents infarcts.
- Therefore, if clopidogrel plus aspirin in combination, or warfarin, is required for other indications (e.g. acute coronary syndrome or pulmonary embolism) the occurrence of stroke is not a contraindication to their use.
- The combination of aspirin 75mg/day and clopidogrel 75mg/day reduces the number of microembolic signals detected on transcranial Doppler studies after a TIA. Some trial evidence (Box 10.5, p.243; also see ☐ Box 10.21, p.274) supports use of the combination in the short term (1 month) after a TIA, albeit inconclusively. It is possible that if the risk of infarction is particularly high early after a TIA, and the risk of intracranial bleeding is more constant over time, then the additional antithrombotic effect may produce a net benefit in this situation. However, there is still an excess of intracranial haemorrhages in the short term.
- For patients with very frequent recurrences, make sure that the diagnosis is right (fits or migraine can deceive even experienced doctors). The combination of aspirin and clopidogrel may be tried in the short term. Anticoagulation, or the combination of aspirin and warfarin, is probably ineffective.
- Coprescribe a proton pump inhibitor in high-risk groups (history of peptic ulcer in the past 10 years, coprescription of corticosteroids or non-steroidal anti-inflammatory drugs). Ibuprofen may diminish the protective effect of aspirin.
- If a patient develops anaemia on aspirin, investigate it (haematinics, upper GI endoscopy, and large bowel investigations if necessary and appropriate).
- There is no benefit in giving aspirin (or other antithrombotics) to people without symptomatic vascular disease (cerebrovascular, coronary, or peripheral), on the basis of risk factors alone.

Box 10.3 Antiplatelet agents prevent strokes and other vascular events: Anti-Thrombotic Trialists collaboration

- The collaboration included 197 trials of antiplatelet therapy vs control (n=136000), 90 comparisons of different antiplatelet regimens (n=77 000), and 17 000 vascular outcome events (MI, stroke, or vascular death), including 4900 strokes.
- Aspirin reduced vascular events with a RR on treatment of 0.75 (95% CI 0.71–0.79), for patients at high risk of vascular disease (>3%/year). Vascular death (RR 0.85, 95% CI 0.81–0.89), and all-cause mortality were reduced.
- Aspirin reduced non-fatal strokes (RR 0.75, 95% CI 0.69–0.81), with no difference between categories of patient treated (prior MI, acute MI, prior stroke or TIA, other high risk).
- Overall RR of any stroke on treatment was 0.78 (95% CI 0.72–0.84). Haemorrhagic strokes increased on treatment (RR 1.22, 95% CI 1.03–1.44), but ischaemic strokes decreased (RR 0.70, 95% CI 0.65–0.76).
- Greater case fatality in haemorrhagic strokes offset the reduction in fatal strokes (RR 0.84, 95% CI 0.70–0.98).
- Disabling strokes and fatal strokes together were reduced (RR 0.76, 95% CI 0.58–0.94).
- Aspirin reduced total vascular events amongst 18 000 patients with a prior history of stroke or TIA (RR 0.78, 95% CI 0.70–0.86). Patients with TIA and completed strokes had the same benefit.
- The effect was regardless of aspirin dose (down to 75mg/day).
- Doses <75mg/day may be less effective than 75–150mg/day, but with current data differences are within the range that might have been expected by chance.
- Benefit continued to be observed into the 2nd and 3rd years of treatment.
- 787 major extracranial bleeds were recorded, RR on treatment 1.6 (95% CI 1.4–1.8).
- Clopidogrel reduced vascular events slightly more than aspirin (RR 0.91, 95% CI 0.83–0.99).
- Healthy people at low risk of vascular events (<1% per year), and people in primary prevention populations (on the basis of vascular risk factors, but without overt vascular disease) did not benefit from aspirin.

British Medical Journal 1994; **308**:81–106.
British Medical Journal 2002; **324**:71–86.
Lancet 2009; **373**:1849–60.

Box 10.4 Aspirin plus dipyridamole for secondary prevention (ESPRIT Trial)

- 2739 patients within 6 months of a TIA (1/3) or non-disabling ischaemic stroke (2/3) were randomized to aspirin (30–325mg) with or without dipyridamole (200mg bd). Mean age 63 years, 16% were >75 years.
- 1068 patients were separately randomized between aspirin and oral anticoagulation (INR 2–3).
- Follow-up was mean 3.5 years for the dipyridamole trial, 4.6 years for the anticoagulation trial. Outcome was combined vascular death, non-fatal stroke, non-fatal MI, and major bleeding.
- RR on aspirin/dipyridamole compared with aspirin were:
  - 0.80 (95% CI 0.66–0.98) for any vascular event or major bleed (13% vs 16%).
  - 0.84 (95% CI 0.64–1.10) for ischaemic stroke (7.0% vs 8.4%).
  - 0.88 (95% CI 0.62–0.83) for all-cause mortality (6.8% vs 7.8%).
- RR on oral anticoagulation compared with aspirin were:
  - 1.02 (95% CI 0.77–1.35) for any vascular event or major bleed (19% vs 18%).
  - 0.76 (95% CI 0.51–1.15) for ischaemic stroke (7.6% vs 10.0%).
  - 2.6 (95% CI 1.5–4.4) for major bleeds.
  - 1.36 (95% CI 0.92–2.01) for all-cause mortality (11% vs 8.3%).
- Patients on dipyridamole therapy discontinued medication more often than those on aspirin monotherapy, mainly because of headache (34% vs 13%).
- The comparison between oral anticoagulants and aspirin/ dipyridamole combination was unfavourable (RR 1.31 95% CI 0.98–1.75).
- The earlier ESPS-2 trial, which randomized 3299 participants, showed identical results. A meta-analysis of both trials, plus four smaller older trials showed an overall RR of 0.82 (95% CI 0.74–0.91) in favour of combined aspirin/dipyridamole therapy.
- Oral anticoagulation was possibly better at averting cerebral ischaemia (in an underpowered analysis), but this was offset by an increased number of bleeds.

Journal of the Neurological Sciences 1996; **143**:1–13.
Lancet 2006; **367**:1665–73.
Lancet Neurology 2007; **6**:115–24.

Box 10.5 Feasibility trial of early intensive anti-platelet drugs or simvastatin after TIA (FASTER)

- 392 patients within 24h of a minor stroke or TIA were randomized in a 2×2 factorial design to clopidogrel 300mg immediately then 75mg/day or placebo, and to simvastatin 40mg immediately and 40mg/day or placebo. All had 81mg aspirin for study duration, with 162mg loading if aspirin naïve.
- Patients were closely followed up for 90 days. There were 33 new ischaemic stroke and 2 haemorrhages, median time to onset 1 day, range 0–62 days. 12 were disabling, 1 fatal.
- 20% stopped taking clopidogrel, 19% stopped taking simvastatin.
- RR on clopidogrel plus aspirin vs aspirin alone were:
  - 0.7 (95% CI 0.3–1.2) for any stroke (7.1% vs 10.8%).
  - 0.7 (95% CI 0.4–1.3) for stroke, MI, or vascular death (8.6% vs 11.9%).
  - 0.7 (95% CI 0.4–1.2) for stroke, TIA, acute coronary syndrome, any death (14.7% vs 21.7%).
- RR on simvastatin were:
  - 1.5 (95% CI 0.8–2.8) for any stroke (10.6% vs 7.3%).
  - 1.3 (95% CI 0.7–2.4) for stroke, MI, or vascular death (11.6% vs 8.8%).
  - 1.1 (95% CI 0.7–1.7) for stroke, TIA, acute coronary syndrome, any death (19.1% vs 17.1%).
- Clopidogrel was associated with two intracranial haemorrhages (about 1%) and four symptomatic extracranial bleeds (vs none in the aspirin only group).

Lancet Neurology 2007; **6**:961–69.

Smoking

- Smoking doubles the risk of both cerebral infarcts and bleeds.
- Risk reduces to near that of never-smokers within 2–5 years of stopping.
- It is never too late to give up.
- Specialist professional or group support, nicotine replacement, varenicline, and bupropion all increase the chances of successfully quitting (5% give up on advice alone, 10–20% with drug treatment). Of the three, varenicline is the most effective. Drugs should only be used if the patient agrees to stop smoking, and should be discontinued if they restart smoking.
- Nicotine replacement delivers less nicotine than continuing to smoke, and is safer than continued smoking in cardiovascular disease and hypertension. Transdermal patches are convenient. Use a 16-h patch to avoid insomnia. Starting dose is determined by number of cigarettes previously smoked per day. Reduce dose every 3 weeks, maximum duration of treatment 10–12 weeks. Other administration routes (chewing gum, nasal spray, sublingual) may help some individuals.
- Many patients successfully use the opportunity of hospitalization for stroke to stop. Discuss and encourage this.
- Stopping smoking is hard, and may take several attempts. Relapse is common. Sympathize, don't blame or stigmatize.
- Withdrawal symptoms include craving, irritability, inability to concentrate, restlessness, hunger, poor sleep, depressed mood, and general malaise.
- The more times you try stopping, the better your chances of ultimate success!

Blood pressure

Principles

- BP is causally related to risk of stroke (both infarcts and bleeds).
- Risk increases 40% for each 10-mmHg increase in systolic BP, although this effect declines somewhat with age.
- BP reduction reduces the risk of cerebral infarcts and bleeds, and ischaemic heart disease, within a few years of treatment. Reduction of BP is important above all else, regardless of which drugs are used (Boxes 10.6 and 10.7).
- Isolated systolic hypertension is as important as combined systolic and diastolic hypertension.
- BP reduction is beneficial regardless of age, although extreme care is required when treating frail people (Box 10.8).
- BP is often raised after a stroke, and will reduce spontaneously over about a week. For secondary prevention start (or increase) drugs after that.
- Do not treat a single, one-off, BP. Clinic readings are often raised. 5min of lying down, followed by a nurse-measured BP, is often better. Ward observations records provide a good guide to 'usual' BP. If in doubt about degree of hypertension, or 'white coat' hypertension, get 24-h ambulatory monitoring.
- The lower the BP, the better, so long as symptomatic hypotension is not induced (postural dizziness or syncope, mainly). Less than 130/80 is suggested for people with diabetes—this should go for anyone with a stroke as well.
- For a preventative intervention, troublesome side effects of treatment are not to be tolerated (you should not sacrifice current well-being for uncertain future benefits).
- BP control will usually be monitored in primary care. Those who can afford it might be encouraged to buy a home BP monitoring machine (under £50 in the UK; search the internet or ask at a pharmacy).
- High BP is usually undertreated in the UK.
- Monotherapy is unlikely to be effective—there are multiple physiological BP control systems, and inhibiting one will often produce counter-regulation in others.
- Use effective doses (but using several agents at low dose is an effective strategy to reduce BP whilst minimizing side effects).

Which drugs?

- Stroke patients often have other things wrong with them, and BP lowering therapy can be tailored to take into account additional benefits, and to avoid particular side effects or complications (Table 10.2).
- Calcium channel blockers (CCBs) may be marginally the best drugs for preventing stroke, but after that there is little to choose between thiazides, ACEIs, or angiotensin receptor blockers (ARBs). Atenolol and alpha-blockers appear to be marginally less effective (Boxes 10.6 and 10.7; ℘ www.thegeorgeinstitute.org/bplttc/results.html).

- CCBs are safe, effective, and cheap. But they can cause troublesome oedema and constipation, and increase heart failure compared with thiazides (Box 10.6).
- Thiazides (bendroflumethazide 2.5mg daily, chlortalidone 25mg daily) are the best established antihypertensive drugs, are cheap, and have the same incidence of side effects as other agents (Box 10.6).
- ACEIs have a good track record in vascular secondary prevention (Boxes 10.6–10.9):
  - They are useful when there is comorbid heart or renal failure, diabetes, or previous MI.
  - A proportion of stroke patients will also have renovascular disease. Check biochemical renal function, and recheck a fortnight after starting. If BP is difficult to control, get a renal artery MRA.
  - The action is probably a class effect. Enalapril, lisinopril, ramipril, and perindopril all have hard end-point (total vascular events) trials supporting their use. Perindopril has the advantage of rapid titration up to its maximum dose and long duration of action, but is relatively expensive.
- ARBs seem to have all the benefits of ACEIs, and avoid the problem of ACEI-induced cough. But they are more expensive.
- Alpha-blockers (e.g. doxazosin MR 4mg od) are useful when there is bladder outflow obstruction due to benign prostatic hyperplasia, or incomplete bladder emptying poststroke. However, in the biggest comparative trial, doxazosin-based treatment prevented fewer cardiovascular events, especially heart failure and stroke, than did treatment based on chlortalidone (Box 10.7).
- Beta-blockers are useful if there is also ischaemic heart disease or heart failure (Box 10.6). However, in a number of trials atenolol performed less well than comparators (thiazides, losartan, ACEIs, CCBs). Atenolol is better than placebo, and differences are small, but is no longer a first-line choice in the absence of a coindication.
- Theoretical benefits of some drugs over others on lipids and glucose tolerance are unimportant in terms of clinical outcomes (even for patients with 'metabolic syndrome').
- Two-thirds of patients will need more than one drug to get adequate control. The British Hypertension Society recommends a stepped approach, although the order in which drugs are added is probably unimportant, regardless of age (Table 10.3). There is a case for using combination products to simplify drug regimens and reduce the numbers of tablets taken, although these have been frowned upon in the past.

Box 10.6 Are some antihypertensive drugs more effective than others?

- A meta-analysis of BP reduction trials, including 108 placebo controlled drug trials, and 46 trials which compared different drugs. Overall, 464 000 participants were randomized.
- Outcome events were 22 000 fatal or non-fatal MIs or sudden cardiac deaths (coronary heart disease [CHD] events) and 12 000 strokes.
- RR on treatment (compared with placebo) were:
  - 0.69 (95% CI 0.62–0.76) for CHD events for people given beta-blockers within a year or two of acute MI.
  - 0.78 (95% CI 0.73–0.83) for CHD events for a 10/5mmHg reduction in BP, regardless of history of prior vascular events.
  - 0.59 (95% CI 0.52–0.67) for strokes for a 10/5mmHg reduction in BP, regardless of history of prior vascular events.
- RR for different drugs, compared with placebo (i.e. indirect comparisons), were:
  - Thiazides: 0.86 (95% CI 0.75–0.98) for CHD events; 0.62 (95% CI 0.53–0.72) for strokes.
  - Beta-blockers: 0.89 (95% CI 0.78–1.02) for CHD events; 0.83 (95% CI 0.70–0.99) for strokes.
  - ACEI: 0.83 (95% CI 0.78–0.89) for CHD events; 0.78 (95% CI 0.66–0.92) for strokes.
  - ARB: 0.86 (95% CI 0.53–1.40) for CHD events; (no data for strokes).
  - CCB: 0.85 (95% CI 0.78–0.92) for CHD events; 0.66 (95% CI 0.58–0.75) for strokes.
  - Any drug: 0.85 (95% CI 0.81–0.89) for CHD events; 0.73 (95% CI 0.66–0.80) for strokes.
- In direct comparisons between drug classes:
  - For CHD prevention all drugs were comparable, within ±10% RR reduction (excluding trials of beta-blockers after acute MI).
  - For stroke prevention, beta-blockers were less good (RR 1.18 95% CI 1.03–1.36) and CCB better (RR 0.91, 95% CI 0.84–0.98) than all other comparator drugs combined.
  - Moderate differences between drug classes (up to 20% RR reduction) for some outcomes could not be excluded.
- Apart from those described, there was little to support differences between drug classes over and above their effect on BP, beyond the random variation expected from one trial to another. Differences between different drugs within classes were also no greater than might be expected by chance.
- Reduced risk was evident within a year of starting treatment. The size of risk reduction was independent of baseline BP (down to 110/70), and was in line with that expected from observational epidemiology on the association between BP and risk, for both stroke and CHD.

British Medical Journal 2009; **338**:b1665.

Box 10.7 Blood pressure-lowering based on different classes of drugs was about equally effective (ALLHAT)

- A comparison of antihypertensive treatment regimens based on chlortalidone (a thiazide diuretic, 12.5–25mg/day, the 'standard' comparator), amlodipine (2.5–10mg/day, a CCB), lisinopril (10–40mg/day, an ACEI) and doxazosin (2–8mg/day, an alpha-blocker).
- To avoid 'contamination' between groups, recommended add-on drugs for inadequate control included atenolol, reserpine, and hydralazine.
- 42 424 patients, >55 years old, with BP >140/90mmHg, and with at least one other cardiovascular risk factor were randomized. 90% were switched from other hypertensive treatments for the trial.
- BP control was less good in the lisinopril group (2mmHg systolic).
- 80% of the chlortalidone and amlodipine group were receiving the study drug or another of the same class after 5 years, as were 70% of the lisinopril patients.
- The doxazosin arm was terminated early after median follow-up of 3.3 years. Compared with chlortalidone there was no difference in the primary outcome (MI plus vascular deaths, RR 1.03, 95% CI 0.90–1.17), or all-cause mortality (RR 1.03, 95% CI 0.90–1.15). However, doxazosin-treated patients had more strokes (RR 1.19, 1.01–1.40), total vascular events (25% vs 22%, RR 1.25, 1.17–1.33), and heart failure (RR 2.04, 1.79–2.32).
- The other comparisons had mean follow-up of 4.9 years. The primary outcome occurred in 11.3–11.5%, with no differences between groups (RR 0.98–0.99, 95% CI ±0.10). All-cause mortality did not differ. Amlodipine treatment was associated with more heart failure (RR1.38, 95% CI 1.25–1.52), and lisinopril treatment was associated with more total vascular events (RR 1.10, 95% CI 1.05–1.15), stroke (RR 1.15, 95% CI 1.02–1.30), and heart failure (RR 1.19, 95% CI 1.07–1.31).
- This trial supports the need to reduce BP using whichever drug classes are required to do so. Excess heart failure in the amlodipine group could be due to the diuretic effect of thiazides, or the negative inotropic effect of amlodipine. The excess strokes in the lisinopril group may have been due to less good BP control.

Journal of the American Medical Association 2000; **283**:1967–75.
Journal of the American Medical Association 2002; **288**:2981–97.

Table 10.2 Coindications, benefits, and common adverse effects of antihypertensive drugs

Drug	Useful coindications and other benefits	Common adverse effects
Thiazides	Less heart failure, can reduce nocturnal polyuria, cheap	Hypokalaemia, hyponatraemia, gout, impotence, glucose intolerance or diabetes. Generally do not coprescribe with loop diuretics
Beta-blockers	Angina, post-MI, heart failure, tachyarrhythmias, anxiety, migraine, cheap	Cold peripheries, fatigue, wheeze, impotence, heart block, heart failure, sleep disturbance, nightmares
CCBs	Angina, tachyarrhythmias	Oedema, constipation, heart failure, headache
ACEIs	Heart failure, post-MI, diabetes, renal failure	Cough, renal failure, angio-oedema, hypotension, especially if dehydrated or aortic stenosis
Alpha-blockers	Prostatic hyperplasia, incomplete bladder emptying	First-dose hypotension, lethargy, rhinitis, stress incontinence in women
Spironolactone	Heart failure	Nausea, diarrhoea, impotence, hyperkalaemia
ARBs	Heart failure	Few side effects, expensive

Table 10.3 British Hypertension Society guidelines on drug combinations

Step		Drug
1	Age <55 years	ACEI or ARB (A)
	Black or age >55 years	Thiazide (D) or CCB (C)
2		A and D, or A and C
3		A, C, D
4		Add an alpha blocker, beta blocker or spironolactone

ℜ http://www.bhsoc.org; ℜ http://www.nice.org.uk

Box 10.8 Hypertension treatment in people over 80 (HYVET)

- 3845 people aged >80 years with sustained systolic BP of >160mmHg (mean 173/91) were randomized to 1.5mg indapamide, or placebo. 2mg or 4mg perindopril, or placebo, was added, if needed, to achieve the target BP of 150/80mmHg. 25% of actively treated participants received indapamide alone.
- 12% had a history of cardiovascular disease, and 6% diabetes. Overall participants were fitter than average for their age, and were not 'frail'.
- After 2 years, mean BP was 15/6mmHg lower in the active-treatment group. Median follow-up was 1.8 years. Fewer serious adverse events were reported in the active-treatment group (19% vs 23%).
- RR on treatment were:
  - 0.70 (95% CI 0.49–1.01) for fatal or nonfatal stroke (12 vs 18 per 1000 person-years).
  - 0.79 (95% CI 0.65–0.96) for all-cause mortality (47 vs 60 per 1000 person-years).
  - 0.66 (95% CI 0.53–0.82) for any cardiovascular event (34 vs 51 per 1000 person-years).
- The trial terminated early, due to an apparent large reduction in stroke, which was not quite so large when the full dataset was analysed. Consequently, it was underpowered for its primary end-point. Results demonstrate that despite the smaller RR of high BP in very old people compared with younger adults, BP reduction, to a target of 150/80mmHg, at least, is beneficial.

New England Journal of Medicine 2008; **358**:1887–98.

Box 10.9 PROGRESS trial: blood pressure reduction prevents stroke recurrence

- 6105 patients who had had a non-disabling stroke or TIA were randomly assigned BP-lowering treatment or placebo, regardless of whether their BP was 'high' or 'normal' (or even 'low'). No lower limit was placed on BP for entry to the trial.
- Active treatment was perindopril (an ACEI) 2mg, increasing to 4mg after 2 weeks, with indapamide (a thiazide) 2.5mg added at the discretion of the investigator. Combination treatment could be pre-specified, and randomization was stratified for this choice.
- BP was reduced by 9/4mmHg on average. Follow-up was 4 years. New stroke was the primary outcome.
- Half of participants were on other BP drugs at the time of randomization. Thus, benefits of the trial treatment were additional to that gained by being on treatment already.
- RR on treatment were:
  - 0.72 (95% CI 0.62–0.83) for any stroke (13.8% vs 10.0%).
  - 0.96 (95% CI 0.82–1.12) for all-cause mortality (10.4% vs 10.0%).
  - 0.76 (95% CI 0.72–0.81) for any major vascular event (15.0% vs 19.8%).
- RR on treatment were greater on combination therapy (mean BP reduction 12/5mmHg) compared with single drug (mean BP reduction 5/3mmHg).
  - For stroke: 0.95 (95% CI 0.77–1.19 i.e. no effect) single drug vs 0.57 (95% CI 0.46–0.70) combined.
  - For major vascular events: 0.96 (95% CI 0.80–1.15) single drug vs 0.60 (95% CI 0.51–0.71) combined.
- Reduced risk on treatment was similar regardless of type of stroke, and initial BP (i.e. reducing 'normal' BP is beneficial).
- The HOPE and EUROPA trials showed similar benefits for patients with high vascular risk or stable ischaemic heart disease treated with ramipril or perindopril.

New England Journal of Medicine 2000; **342**:145–53.
Lancet 2001; **358**:1033–41.
British Medical Journal 2002; **324**:699–702.
Lancet 2003; **362**:782–8.

Cholesterol

- For many years it appeared that cholesterol concentration was not a risk factor for stroke. This was possibly because of inability to separate ischaemic stroke (risk increases with higher cholesterol) from haemorrhagic stroke (risk decreases with higher cholesterol) in older studies.
- In prevention trials of statins for people with ischaemic heart disease, incidence of stroke was reduced by 31% (as well as the benefits in preventing other vascular disease).
- The Heart Protection Study treated all patients (with simvastatin 40mg or placebo) deemed at high risk, by virtue of a previous vascular event, diabetes, or multiple vascular risk factors, and regardless of their initial cholesterol. There was a 25% reduction in vascular events, including amongst patients who had had a previous stroke (Box 10.10). Other trials have replicated this (Boxes 10.11 and 10.12).
- HMG CoA reductase inhibitors (statins) are the most useful drugs. Dietary advice is wise (weight loss, low cholesterol and animal fat, functional foods e.g. Benecol®), and effects are additional to those of drugs, but statins are considerably more powerful than the effect of diet alone.
- However, statins increase risk of bleeding and should be avoided after intracerebral haemorrhage (Box 10.12).
- Simvastatin is well proven, reduces cholesterol by up to 50%, and is cheap. Start at 40mg. Myositis is a rare but important complication (measure creatine kinase if worried). Rosuvastatin and atorvastatin reduce cholesterol by an additional 10% or so.
- Ezetimibe (10mg od) reduces cholesterol by another 25%. It can be added to statins, or used alone if a statin is not tolerated.
- Aggressive cholesterol lowering (to a target low-density lipoprotein-cholesterol [LDL-C] <1.8mmol/L) appears to cause regression of atheromatous plaques. Some (albeit incomplete) evidence suggests this is translated into fewer strokes or other cardiovascular events.

Box 10.10 Heart Protection Study (HPS)

- Participants were 20 536 people aged 40–80 years at high risk of vascular death by virtue of a prior vascular event (including 3280 who had had a stroke), diabetes, or treated hypertension in men >65 years old, and with a total cholesterol >3.5mmol/L.
- They were given simvastatin 40mg a day or placebo, and followed-up for 5 years.
- On average, 85% of the intervention group took their drug, and 17% of the control group were given an out-of-trial statin. Total cholesterol was reduced on average by 1.2mmol/L (LDL-C reduced by 1.0mmol/L), but the difference between intervention and control dropped from 1.7mmol/L in the 1st year, to 0.8mmol/L in the 5th year.
- RR on treatment were:
  - 0.87 (95% CI 0.81–0.94) for all-cause mortality (12.9% vs 14.7%).
  - 0.76 (95% CI 0.72–0.81) for any major vascular event (19.8% vs 25.2%).
  - 0.75 (95% CI 0.66–0.85) for any stroke (and TIA) (4.3% vs 5.7%).
- There was no increase in haemorrhagic strokes (although numbers were few and this was statistically uncertain), nor fatal or more severe strokes.
- There were no differences in effect according to the presence or absence of CHD, prior disease category that allowed entry to the trial, age, sex, initial cholesterol level, or any other variable, including other preventative drug treatments. This indicated that the effects are additive to those of the other treatments.
- Myositis was very rare (10 simvastatin vs 4 placebo).

Lancet 2002; **360**:7–22

Box 10.11 Meta-analysis of cholesterol-lowering treatment effects

- Data from 14 randomized trials of statins, including 90 056 participants, about half with pre-existing CHD. Mean follow-up was 5 years, with 8186 deaths, 14 348 vascular events, 2957 strokes, and 5103 cancers recorded.
- Mean baseline LDL-C was 3.8mmol/L; mean reduction at 1 year 1.1mmol/L; mean reduction at 5 years 0.8mmol/L.
- RR on treatment, per mmol/L reduction in LDL-C were:
  - 0.88 (95% CI 0.84–0.91) for all-cause mortality (8.5% vs 9.7%).
  - 0.77 (95% CI 0.74–0.80) for MI (7.4% vs 9.8%).
  - 0.83 (95% CI 0.78–0.88) for stroke (3.0% vs 3.7%).
  - 0.78 (95% CI 0.70–0.87) for ischaemic stroke (2.8% vs 3.4%).
  - 0.79 (95% CI 0.77–0.81) for any major vascular event (14.1% vs 17.8%).
- NNT are 48 fewer major vascular events (8 strokes) per 1000 treated for those with pre-existing CHD, and 25 (5 strokes) per 1000 without pre-existing CHD.
- Reduction in vascular events varied with LDL-C reduction achieved, but no other variable influenced treatment effect (including initial LDL-C, diabetes, prior vascular disease, or age).
- Benefit was evident within the 1st year of treatment, but was larger in the 2nd and subsequent years.
- Statins did not increase cancer risk (RR 1.0, 95% CI 0.90–1.06). Effects on intracerebral haemorrhage were uncertain, as data were consistent with both a 20% reduction and a 40% increase (RR 1.05, 95% CI 0.78–1.41).
- Rhabdomyolysis was seen in 0.023% (statin) vs 0.015% (control).

Lancet 2005; **366**:1267–78.

Box 10.12 High-dose atorvastatin after stroke or TIA in the absence of ischaemic heart disease (SPARCL)

- 4731 patients within 6 months of a stroke or TIA, in whom there was no evidence of ischaemic heart disease, were randomized to atorvastatin 80mg or placebo. Mean follow-up was 4.9 years. Primary end-point was fatal or non-fatal stroke.
- Out-of-trial statins were used in 25% of the placebo group and 11% of the atorvastatin group. Mean difference between groups was 1.6mmol/L for total cholesterol, and 1.4mmo/L for LDL-C.
- RR on treatment were:
  - 0.84 (95% CI 0.71–0.99) for fatal or non-fatal stroke (11.2% vs 13.1%).
  - 0.80 (95% CI 0.69–0.92) for major cardiovascular events (14.1% vs 17.2%).
  - 1.66 (95% CI 1.08–2.55) for haemorrhagic stroke (2.3% vs 1.4%).
  - 1.0 (95% CI 0.0.82–1.21) for all-cause mortality (9.1% vs 8.9%).
- These results are broadly in line those of other statin trials. The increase in bleeds may reflect an antithrombotic effect of statins, and cautions against use in intracerebral haemorrhage.

New England Journal of Medicine 2006; **355**:549–60.

Homocysteine

Homocysteine level is associated with stroke and heart attack in observational studies. Folic acid and vitamins B12 and B6 supplementation lowers homocysteine by about 30%. Unfortunately, giving these vitamins has no effect on heart attack or all-cause mortality, and inconclusive effects on risk of stroke (one trial suggested a 25% reduction in stroke, others no effect).

Lifestyle changes

- The evidence for the effectiveness of interventions to promote lifestyle changes is limited (Box 10.13). But that may be due to difficulty in sustaining lifestyle changes of a sufficient intensity for people not used to them, and demonstrating any effects experimentally. There is little doubt that, for example, vegetarians, those who maintain ideal body weight, or who exercise regularly, have fewer heart attacks and strokes.
- Effects often wane over a year or so—advice will need repeating.
- Changes help promote a sense of taking control of responsibility for health. They should all be discussed with patients who survive with no more than mild to moderate disability.
- BP can be reduced (in approximate order of efficacy), by:
  • Weight loss.
  • Reducing heavy alcohol intake.
  • Eating more fruit and vegetables.
  • Restricting salt intake.

None of these approaches the efficacy of drug treatment.

- Suggest moderate exercise, for at least 20min, at least three times a week, preferably daily. Try to build this into the daily routine (getting to work, work, stairs, housework, gardening, shopping).
- BP reduction from weight loss of 5kg is about 4.4/3.6mmHg. Weight loss has vascular benefits beyond those on BP and cholesterol, and relief of stress on arthritic knees. Aim for 5–10% over 3 months. This is realistically achievable and sustainable. Weight loss requires eating less, in particular energy (calories: fat, carbohydrate, alcohol), and in practice cannot be achieved by exercise alone. When you starve you lose both fat and muscle; exercise is required in addition to prevent muscle loss.
- Reduce alcohol intake to standard 'sensible' limits (men <21 units/week, women <14 units/week, half this in people >75 years old, abstention for people with a history of alcohol problems; 1 unit = 10g ethanol, 1 small glass wine, single measure spirits, half pint/250mL beer).

Box 10.13 Trials of lifestyle changes

- A 2×2 factorial trial (TOPH II) of weight loss, dietary sodium restriction, or both, was carried out in 2382 participants with 'high normal' BP (mean 128/86mmHg), who were slightly overweight:
  - Mean weight reduction in the intervention group compared with the usual care group was 4.5kg at 6 months, and 2kg at 3 years.
  - Mean sodium excretion was less in the sodium reduction group compared with the usual care group, by 50mmol/day after 6 months, and 40mmol/day after 3 years, but only 35mmol/day after 6 months and 25mmol/day after 3 years in the combined group.
  - Mean BP at 6 months reduced 3.7/2.7mmHg in the weight loss group, 2.9/1.6mmHg in the sodium reduction group, and 4.0/2.8mmHg in the combined group, but this waned to 1.3/0.9mmHg after 3 years. Over 4 years there was a 20% reduction in the incidence of 'hypertension' (BP >140/90mmHg) in both intervention groups.
- 77% of 3126 participants randomized in both TOPH II and the prior TOPH I trial were followed up 10–15 years later. Intervention had been for 18–48 months only.
- A diet questionnaire revealed that the intervention group were substantially more likely to be aware of dietary salt and to avoid salty foods.
- RR in the sodium intake reduction group were:
  - 0.75 (95% CI 0.57–0.99) for all cardiovascular events (7.5% vs 9.0%).
  - 0.81 (95% CI 0.52–1.27) for all-cause mortality (2.3% vs 2.6%).
- Another trial studied 201 men with high normal BP, and intervened to achieve a 2.7kg mean weight reduction, 25% reduced mean sodium intake, and 30% decreased alcohol intake:
  - Mean BP reduced 2.0/1.9mmHg. RR of developing 'hypertension' in the intervention group compared with control was 0.42, 95% CI 0.21–0.83 (19.2% vs 8.8%).
- A 3rd trial randomized 459 participants between control diet, fruit and vegetable rich diet, and a fruit and vegetable rich, low fat diet:
  - Initial mean BP was 131/85mmHg. The intervention diets reduced this over 8 weeks by 2.8/1.1 and 5.5/3.0mmHg. Amongst hypertensive subjects mean reductions were up to 11/6mmHg.
- Intervention was hard work, entailing intensive advice and support from dieticians, doctors, psychologists, and counsellors, individually and in groups, including involvement of family members, up to weekly initially, and 1–2-monthly after that. In the 3rd trial, all meals were prepared centrally.
- Lifestyle modification does reduce BP. Changes are difficult, but may be maintained over long periods of time. BP reductions are small compared with those that can be achieved with drugs.

Journal of the American Medical Association 1989; **262**:1801–7.
Archives of Internal Medicine 1997; **157**:657–67.
New England Journal of Medicine 1997; **336**:1117–24.
Archives of Internal Medicine 2008; **168**:713–20.

Hormone replacement therapy and the contraceptive pill

- Combined oestrogen–progestogen HRT increases the risk of stroke and should be avoided unless there are troublesome menopausal symptoms (certainly after a stroke).
- The combined oral contraceptive pill also increases the relative risk of stroke, but the absolute risks are low in young women. If someone has a stroke on the pill, alternative contraception should be used (progesterone-only pill, intrauterine contraceptive device, barrier methods, or sterilization).

Carotid stenosis

- Patients with anterior circulation stroke, who survive with no more than mild to moderate disability, and who would be willing to have an operation, should be screened for carotid stenosis on the symptomatic side by duplex ultrasound scanning, MRA or CTA.
- Most lacunar strokes are not be caused by carotid atheroma, but distinguishing them from partial anterior circulation strokes is not always reliable. Moreover, some lacunar strokes may be embolic.
- Note that there are different systems for grading degree of carotid stenosis.
- Patients with >70% stenosis (European Carotid Surgery Trial [ECST] method, >50% North American Symptomatic Carotid Endarterectomy Trial [NASCET] method) benefit overall from carotid endarterectomy, so long as the surgeon has an audited average complication rate (death or disabling stroke) of <5% (Box10.14).
- For every 20 operations done, 1 patient has a stroke perioperatively, and 4 patients avoid a stroke over the next 5 years. These figures vary with degree of stenosis and other risk factors, however.
- There is a 1 in 100 chance of death, and a 1 in 40 chance of a cranial nerve palsy (hoarse voice, usually recovers). These odds should be explained to the patient.
- Surgery should be done quickly (within 48h of assessment if possible). Surgery performed within 2 weeks has NNT=5 to prevent one stroke in 5 years. For surgery performed after 12 weeks NNT is 125 (i.e. essentially worthless).
- Surgery can be done under local or general anaesthetic.
- Some groups benefit more than others (men, those >75 years, more severe stenosis, completed stroke rather than TIA, hemispheric rather than ocular TIA). This information may help in decision making: importantly, older people should not be excluded from considering surgery on grounds of age alone.
- Carotid angioplasty and stenting is an alternative to surgical endarterectomy, where there is local neuroradiological expertise. Trials have failed to show that it is superior to surgery, and outcomes may be worse (Box10.15). Local complications (cranial nerve palsies) and bleeding complications are fewer. But there is a greater chance of recurrence of stenosis than with surgery. Techniques are still evolving, and, in general, stenting should be reserved for trials, where lesions are technically inaccessible, unsuitable for surgery, or where anaesthetic risk is high.
- Asymptomatic carotid stenosis (often the other side when a potentially symptomatic artery is investigated) is not generally an indication for carotid surgery. Two trials demonstrated a reduction in stroke rate following operation (from 10% to 5% over 5 years, with a very low perioperative complication rate of 2%). The baseline risk of stroke attributable to asymptomatic stenosis is low. You need to do 100 operations to prevent one stroke in a year.

Box 10.14 Carotid surgery trials

- Two large-scale randomized trials studied the efficacy of carotid endarterectomy in preventing strokes—the ECST and the NASCET. Results (on 6092 patients) have been pooled and reanalysed.
- Follow-up was 1–167 months, mean 65 months, giving 35 000 person-years of follow-up, and 1265 patients experiencing a stroke or death.
- 10% were >75 years. 43% had a stroke, 38% TIA, and 19% ocular events. All were randomized within 6 months of the qualifying event, 41% within 1 month.
- ECST and NASCET adopted different conventions for describing degree of internal carotid stenosis on angiograms. The reanalysis adopted the NASCET convention. NASCET 50% is ECST 65%, and NASCET 70% is ECST 82%. 'Near-occlusion' (underfilling of the distal internal carotid) was a separate category.
- Comparison was between surgery (most performed within 14 days of randomization) plus best medical management, vs medical management alone.
- Outcomes included any stroke lasting >24h. Disabling stroke was defined as a Rankin score of 3 or more (needing help from others).
- Surgery was associated with a perioperative (30 days) risk (1.1% deaths, 7.1% death or stroke). Medical management has a steady accrual of risk over time. A single RR cannot describe findings adequately.
- Absolute risk reductions with surgery, for any stroke or operative death after 5 years were:
  - −0.1% (95% CI −10% to +10%) for near occlusion (22% surgical vs 22% medical).
  - 15% (95% CI 10–21%) for 70–99% stenosis (16% vs 31%).
  - 8% (95% CI 3–13%) for 50–69% stenosis (19% vs 27%).
  - 3% (95% CI −2 to 7%) for 30–49% stenosis (21% vs 24%).
  - −3% (95% CI −6 to +1%) for <30% stenosis (18% vs 15%).
- Absolute risk reductions with surgery, for disabling or fatal ipsilateral stroke after 5 years or operative stroke or death, were:
  - −2% (95% CI −9% to +4%) for near occlusion (8% surgical vs 6% medical).
  - 7% (95% CI 4–10%) for 70–99% stenosis (3% vs 10%).
  - 2% (95% CI 0–5%) for 50–69% stenosis (3% vs 5%).
  - 0 (95% CI −2 to +3%) for 30–49% stenosis (5% vs 5%).
  - −2% (95% CI −4 to 0%) for <30% stenosis (4% vs 2%).
- NNT for 50–69% stenosis is 13 over 5 years, but the reduction in disabling stroke was very small. NNT is 6 for 70–99% stenosis.

Lancet 2003; **361**:107–16.

Box 10.15 Endarterectomy vs stenting in symptomatic severe carotid stenosis (EVA-3S)

- 527 patients with symptomatic 60–99% carotid stenosis were randomly assigned to angioplasty and stenting or endarterectomy, mostly with distal cerebral protection. Randomization was within 120 days of symptoms, and intervention was within 2 weeks of randomization. The trial was designed to demonstrate non-inferiority, and was terminated early due to futility and safety concerns.
- Follow-up was at 30 days and 6 months. Primary outcome was any stroke or death.
- At 30 days RR of stenting were:
  - 2.5 (95% CI 1.2–5.1) for any stroke or death (9.6% vs 3.9%).
  - 2.2 (95% CI 0.7–7.2) for disabling stroke or death (3.4% vs 1.5%).
- Risk of any stroke or death was reduced to 7.9% by use of a cerebral protection device. Cranial nerve injuries were fewer with stenting (7.7% vs 1.1%), and length of hospital stay was shorter.
- At 6 months risks of any stroke or death were 11.7% vs 6.1%.

New England Journal of Medicine 2006; **355**:1660–71.

Atrial fibrillation

- Risk of stroke is increased 5-fold in the presence of AF (paroxysmal or sustained). Risks are higher in the presence of other risk factors, including heart failure and hypertension, and with increasing age (Box 10.16).
- Rhythm control (electrically or chemically restoring sinus rhythm) does not reliably reduce risk of stroke (possibly because of high AF recurrence rates).
- There are several systems to quantify risk:
  - The CHADS$_2$ score (Box10.17). Simple, but underestimates risk for someone in AF who has had a first stroke or TIA as their only additional risk factor. No better than modest accuracy in risk prediction, overall.
  - The UK NICE algorithm (Box10.18) is based on descriptions of risk factor combinations, rather than scores.
  - The Framingham score (see ☐ Appendix 14, p.348) is similar, with more gradations for age and BP level.
- Risk of recurrence is about 5% in the 4 weeks after a stroke for someone in AF, but early anticoagulation does not produce net benefit.
- Warfarin treatment (INR 2–3) reduces the risk by two-thirds in the longer term. But this is at the cost of the inconvenience of having to be monitored, about 2–4%/year chance of severe bleeding (requiring admission or transfusion), and up to 50% chance of minor bleeding per year (bruising, nosebleeds, cuts and abrasions) (Boxes 10.19 and 10.20).
- Commence warfarin 1–2 weeks after stroke onset, after intracranial haemorrhage has been excluded by early CT scanning.
- Aspirin treatment is less effective, reducing strokes by one-fifth, but at considerably less risk (0.5% per year chance of GI bleeding).
- Estimate absolute stroke risk for your patient, using CHADS$_2$, NICE, or Framingham risk scores. Use this to estimate the absolute risk reduction and NNT. This can help in counselling and decision making about warfarin, and may aid compliance. Patients with AF whose stroke risk exceeds 4% per year should usually be anticoagulated in the absence of contraindications, but individual patients may choose otherwise.
- For example, a patient in AF with a 12% stroke risk per year will have this reduced to 9% with aspirin, and 4% with warfarin. NNT are 12 per year for warfarin and 33 for aspirin.
- Younger patients with AF and *no other risk factors* are unlikely to benefit from warfarin, perhaps counterintuitively. Risk of stroke for patients who are <75 years of age without prior stroke or TIA is 1–2% per year (if given aspirin), and they do not benefit sufficiently from anticoagulation to warrant its use for primary stroke prevention.
- Reasons for not giving warfarin include history of intracerebral bleeding, likely poor compliance or anticipated problems with monitoring, possible systemic bleeding (e.g. unexplained iron deficiency anaemia), frequent falls, and patient choice (Box 10.19).
- The key to good decision making is simple and clear explanation of the risk/benefit ratio (not easy), and informed patient choice.

- Adding aspirin to warfarin is of no net benefit, but increases bleeding risks. The combination may be used if a patient also has acute coronary syndrome. Warfarin is superior to the combination of aspirin and clopidogrel. Aspirin plus clopidogrel is marginally more effective than aspirin alone (11% RR reduction for combined vascular events) at the cost of marginally more intracerebral bleeds and a doubling of all major bleeds (2% vs 1.3%).

Box 10.16 Stroke risk in AF

- Pooled data from prevention trials were used to derive risk models for stroke in AF.
- Age, history of hypertension, and previous stroke or TIA all increased risk of stroke. Annual risks for age <65, 65–75, and >75 years with no risk factors were 1.0%, 4.3%, and 3.5%. With one or more additional risk factors, the risks were 4.9%, 5.7%, and 8.1% per year.
- Another study identified heart failure, hypertension, and previous thromboembolism as risk factors. Risks were 2.5%/year if none of the factors was present, 7.2%/year for one factor, 17.6%/year for two or three factors.
- In addition echocardiographic global left ventricular dysfunction, and left atrial size >4.7cm were independent risk factors, with annual risks for none, 1 or 2, and three or more of these factors of 1.0%, 6%, and 18.6%.
- The same data were used to derive the CHADS$_2$ score.

Archives of Internal Medicine 1994; **154**:1449–57.
Journal of the American Medical Association 2003; **290**:1049–56.

Box 10.17 The CHADS$_2$ score for stroke risk in AF

1 point each for presence of:
- Congestive heart failure (active within the past 100 days).
- History of hypertension (treated or not).
- Age 75 years or older.
- Diabetes mellitus.

and, 2 points for:
- History of stroke or TIA.

Total points are summed:
- 0 is low risk; 1–2 is moderate risk; and 3–6 is high risk.
- In a clinical population, without anticoagulant therapy, stroke rates were:

Score	0	1	2	3	4	5	6
% risk/yr	1.9	2.8	4.0	5.9	8.5	12.5	18.2
95% CI	1.2–3.0	2.0–3.8	3.1–5.1	4.6–7.3	6.3–11.1	8.2–17.5	10.5–27.4

- Note that if a patient has a stroke or TIA as their only risk factor (apart from AF), they have a CHADS$_2$ score of 2, incorrectly categorizing them as moderate risk. They are at high risk for both mortality and recurrent stroke.

Journal of the American Medical Association 2001; **285**:2864–70.

Box 10.18 NICE guidelines for antithrombotic therapy in nonvalvular AF

Assess risk, and reassess regularly.
- High risk (risk of stroke=8–12%/year):
  - Patients with previous TIA or ischaemic stroke.
  - Patients aged >75 with hypertension, diabetes, or vascular disease.
  - Patients with clinical evidence of valve disease, heart failure, or impaired left ventricular function on echocardiography.
  - *Treatment:* give warfarin (target INR 2–3) if no contraindications.
- Moderate risk (risk of stroke =4%/year):
  - Patients <65 with hypertension, diabetes, ischaemic heart disease, or peripheral vascular disease.
  - Patients >65 with no high risk factors.
  - *Treatment:* either warfarin (INR 2–3) or aspirin 75–300mg daily. Multiple risk factors increase stroke risk, and potential benefit of warfarin. Echocardiography may help refine risk.
- Low risk (risk of stroke =1%/year):
  - Patients aged <65 with no history of embolism, hypertension, diabetes, or other clinical risk factors.
  - *Treatment:* aspirin 75–300 mg daily.

Echocardiography is not needed for routine risk assessment but refines clinical risk stratification in moderate or severe left ventricular dysfunction. A large atrium per se is not an independent risk factor in multivariate analyses.

NICE guideline 2006;
🖱 www.nice.org.uk/nicemedia/pdf/cg036fullguideline.pdf

Box 10.19 Patients at high risk of bleeding with warfarin

Groups with higher than average risk of bleeding on warfarin:
- Age >75 years (RR of bleeding increases 1.5 per 10 years over 40).
- Uncontrolled hypertension (systolic BP >180mmHg or diastolic BP >100mmHg).
- Alcohol excess (acute or chronic), liver disease.
- Cerebrovascular disease and ischaemic heart disease (including leukoaraiosis).
- Bleeding lesions (e.g. GI blood loss, intracerebral haemorrhage, undiagnosed anaemia).
- Bleeding tendency (coagulation defects, thrombocytopenia).
- Concomitant use of non-steroidal anti-inflammatory drugs.
- Poor drug compliance or poor monitoring clinic attendance.
- High target INR, unstable INR, INR >3.

Note:
- Paradoxically, many risk factors for anticoagulation-related bleeding are also risk factors for thromboembolism in AF. Consider the balance of risks.
- Patients who fall are at greater risk of subdural haematoma and trauma-related bleeding.
- Patients with more than mild cognitive impairment may forget medication, may duplicate doses if they forget they have already taken it, may forget precautions and contraindications, may not attend for monitoring, may fall, and may have leukoaraiosis. However, if adequate support and supervision are available (usually from families) there is no absolute bar to use of anticoagulant drugs.

British Medical Journal 2002; **325**:828–31.
℗ www.nice.org.uk

Box 10.20 Anticoagulation or aspirin in patients with AF

- The European Atrial Fibrillation Study randomized 1007 patients, with a recent stroke or TIA and AF, to aspirin 300mg, warfarin anti-coagulation, or placebo, and a further 2338 patients for whom antico-agulation was contraindicated, to aspirin or placebo.
- RR on warfarin were:
  - 0.53 (95% CI 0.36–0.79) for combined vascular death, stroke, MI, or peripheral embolism (8%/year vs 17%/year).
  - 0.82 (95% CI 0.54–1.26) for all-cause mortality (8%/year vs 9%/year).
  - 0.34 (95% CI 0.20–0.57) for stroke (4%/year vs 12%/year).
- There was no waning of treatment effect with time.
- Warfarin was more effective than aspirin (RR 0.60, 0.41–0.87, NNT 19), and aspirin was probably more effective than placebo (RR 0.83, 0.65–1.05, NNT 25).
- Major bleeds were 2.8% per year for warfarin, 0.9% per year for aspirin, and 0.7% per year for placebo.
- These RR are similar to those from pooled data in primary preven-tion studies (participants with AF without prior stroke)
  - 0.32 (95% CI 0.21–0.50) for warfarin vs placebo.
  - 0.79 (95% CI 0.62–1.0) for aspirin (75–325mg/d) vs placebo.
- A trial comparing warfarin with aspirin 75mg/day in people over 75 (BAFTA) confirmed risks and benefits for this age group. RR on warfarin were:
  - 0.48 (95% CI 0.28–0.80), for fatal or disabling ischaemic or haem-orrhagic stroke, or systemic emboli (1.8%/year vs 3.8%/year)
  - 0.87 (95% CI 0.43–1.73) for extracranial haemorrhage (1.4%/year vs 1.6%/year).
- Risks of major haemorrhage rose with age for both treatments, to 3%/year in people aged >85 years.
- Overall risks for patients on warfarin were minimized at an INR of 2–3.

Lancet 1993; **342**:1255–62.
Archives of Internal Medicine 1994; **154**:1449–57.
Archives of Internal Medicine 1997; **157**:1237–40.
Lancet 2007; **370**:493–503.

Other cardioembolism

- Anticoagulation with warfarin is also indicated for patients who are within 3 months of acute MI, have mitral stenosis, a mechanical prosthetic heart valve, dilated cardiomyopathy, echocardiographically demonstrated mural thrombus, or presumed paradoxical embolism via a patent foramen ovale (PFO), and in whom it is not otherwise contra-indicated.
- Patients with cryptogenic ischaemic stroke who have substantial shunting demonstrated on Valsalva manoeuvre during bubble contrast echocardiographyy, and especially if an atrial septal aneurysm is demonstrated (Box 1.1), can be considered for percutaneous PFO closure.

Pragmatics and compliance

It is not uncommon to see patients admitted to hospital taking 10 or 15 different drugs. Evidence suggests that compliance on the 4th drug is 50%. But you don't know which the 4th drug is.

Help improve compliance if you can.
- Simplify the drug regimen as far as possible:
  - Be sure that each drug is necessary (diuretics, analgesics, sedatives, hypnotics, and laxatives, in particular, should be reviewed critically).
  - Use once-a-day drugs or formulations whenever possible.
  - Use fixed-dose combinations if these are available and suitable.
- If you stop or start drugs during a hospital admission, especially an unusual drug or one used for an unusual indication, explicitly tell the GP in the discharge summary or clinic letter, so that stopped drugs are not inadvertently restarted, or useful drugs stopped during a routine drug review.
- Know if a particular drug is prone to side effects and find out if those effects are occurring. This is a particular issue with loop diuretics causing urinary frequency, urgency, and incontinence in older people, who then often don't take them. For most preventative treatments side effects are unacceptable (you cause a problem now to prevent something that may never happen—and often the odds are usually that it will never happen).
- Make remembering what tablets to take when as easy to take as possible:
  - Ensure patients understand their drugs, know what they are for, and when to take them. Nurses and pharmacists can help here.
  - Explain drug changes as you make them. Some patients are bemused and upset by apparently random stopping and starting of drugs on ward rounds.
  - Self-administration of drugs whilst in hospital helps with familiarity, gives practice, and can alert staff to patients who cannot take drugs reliably.
  - On discharge, write down what to take when.
  - Use 'dosette' boxes or commercial blister pack services, if necessary (from retail pharmacists—at a cost).

- Enlist support from relatives to supervise tablet taking.
- Social Services home care will often prompt to take tablets, but will not usually administer them.
- You can assume that patients in residential or nursing homes will have medication administered reliably.
- Stroke patients may not be able to open child-resistant containers. Check, and provide alternatives if necessary.

Neurovascular or transient ischaemic attack clinics

One or more TIAs precede about a quarter of completed strokes. The rate of recurrent TIA or stroke after a first TIA (or minor stroke) is:

- 10% within a week.
- 13% within a month.
- 18% within 3 months.

A third of these are fatal or disabling. After that, annual rate of stroke is 5% and MI 2.5%. Early risk is 3-fold higher if the TIA or stroke is caused by large artery disease, and 5-fold lower if lacunar.

Since risk is highest in the first 48h, rapid access (same day or within days) to a clinic is necessary for investigation of TIA or minor non-disabling stroke (Box 10.21). If this is not possible, admission to hospital is in the patient's best interests.

Box 10.21 Fast-track TIA services

- Management and outcomes of TIA were studied before and after establishment of an urgent assessment and treatment clinic, within a prospective, population-based, stroke incidence study. The new clinic replaced an existing daily clinic, which already represented better care than usual in the UK at the time.
- Drug therapy (antiplatelet/anticoagulant, BP, and cholesterol lowering) was initiated from the clinic rather than subsequently in primary care. Half of patients were already on antiplatelet drugs at referral, and a third were on statins. Patients seen within 48h or deemed at high risk, and not in AF, had a CT head scan, and were given both aspirin and clopidogrel for 30 days.
- Primary outcome was risk of stroke within 90 days.
- Of 620 patients referred for assessment, 95% were referred to the study clinic. Delay in patients seeking medical attention was identical in both periods, but median delay to assessment fell from 3 (interquartile range [IQR] 2–5) days, to <1 (IQR 0–3) day, and median delay to first prescription of treatment fell from 20 (IQR 8–53 days) to 1 (IQR 0–3) day.
- RR after establishment of the fast-track clinic was:
  - 0.20 (95% CI 0.08–0.49) for new stroke within 90 days (10.3% vs 2.1%).
  - 0.30 (0 95% CI 0.15–0.59) for stroke, MI, or death within 90 days (11.9% vs 3.6%).
- Results were the same for both minor stroke and TIA, and did not vary with age (including those >80 years).
- In the fast-track clinic group, BP was 6/5mmHg lower at 1 month follow-up. Carotid surgery was performed in 5%, and was substantially quicker (within 7 days in 40%). No changes in referral pattern could explain the differences in outcome.

Lancet 2007; **370**:1432–1438.

Diagnosis

Confirming (or refuting) the diagnosis is the first function of a TIA clinic. The diagnosis and differential diagnoses of cerebrovascular disorders were described in 📖 Chapter 1 (p.1 and p.30). Many non-specific or transient symptoms need an explanation. The following problems in isolation are not due to TIA:

- Confusion or forgetfulness.
- Dizziness or light-headedness.
- Blackouts or syncope.
- Falls.
- Incontinence.
- Generalized weakness or sensory symptoms.

Neurological features, present in isolation, not suggestive of TIA, include:

- Paraparesis or quadriparesis.
- Visual hallucinations (might occur due to lesions in the occipital, parietal, or temporal lobe, but more commonly seen in delirium or Lewy body dementia).
- Dysarthria.
- Vertigo (ischaemically-induced *isolated* vertigo is possible but unusual).
- Dysphagia.
- Amnesia.
- Diplopia.
- Hearing loss.

TIA is suggested when there is:

- Sudden onset, transient focal features (e.g. face or limb weakness, aphasia, monocular blindness).
- A combination of features such as diplopia, dysarthria, and dysphagia of sudden onset which suggest brain stem ischaemia.

Risk stratification

Diagnosing TIA is difficult, and ideally all suspected cases should be assessed by a specialist. Even then, clinicians can disagree as to whether a TIA has occurred. The demand for assessment of a variety of non-specific symptoms is high, and in some places no more than 1 in 5 patients seen actually has had a TIA.

The 7-point ABCD2 score (Box 10.22) can be used to prioritize patients according to risk. No doubt this partly works by identifying patients with true TIA. It also tells us that people who have brief or atypical symptoms are generally at low risk, which is a cause for reassurance in difficult cases.

7-day risk is:

- Virtually zero for a score of 0.
- 6% for a score of 4.
- 12% for a score of 6.

Early risk after amaurosis fugax and for pure sensory symptoms is low, but that after posterior circulation TIA is relatively high.

Most conditions being mistaken for TIA have a benign prognosis, including transient global amnesia and uncharacterised dizziness. However, one report found that 'non-focal transient neurological attacks' had an identical prognosis for subsequent stroke as did TIA. Symptoms included transient sensory symptoms, drowsiness, loss of consciousness, unsteadiness, non-rotatory dizziness, positive visual phenomena, bilateral weakness, and malaise that had well-defined sudden onset and full recovery within 24h.

Risk can also be stratified on aetiological grounds. 3-month recurrent stroke rates are:
- Large artery atherothrombosis 20%.
- Cardioembolism 12%.
- Undetermined 5%.
- Small-vessel disease 1.5%.

Of note, if no cause can be determined then recurrence rate is relatively low.

Box 10.22 ABCD2 system for risk stratification after TIA

- Age >65 years: 1 point.
- BP ≥140/90mmHg: 1 point.
- Clinical features, unilateral weakness: 2 points; speech impairment without weakness: 1 point.
- Duration: ≥60min 2 points; 10–59min 1 point.
- Diabetes mellitus: 1 point.

The table gives the risk of stroke after TIA. One-third of these are disabling	High risk	Medium risk	Low risk
ABCD2 score	6–7	4–5	0–3
2-day risk	8.1%	4.1%	1.0%
7-day risk	12%	5.9%	1.2%
90-day risk	18%	9.8%	3.1%

Lancet 2007; **369**:283–92.

Investigations

Carotid duplex scanning

TIA clinics should have immediate access to carotid duplex scanning (or MRA or CTA). It is sensible to screen out people who have not had an anterior circulation TIA clinically, or had bleeds on neuroimaging, and possibly those who would not want an operation if offered it (although knowing you have a tight stenosis might be a factor in deciding). If a tight stenosis is detected on duplex ultrasound, this may be followed up with MR, CT, or other angiography, depending on individual surgeons' preferences, to confirm the stenosis and look for distal vascular disease that might complicate or contraindicate surgery. The pick-up rate from duplex scanning is not high, however—only about 1 in 10 people with a recent TIA will have a 50–99% ipsilateral stenosis, of whom about 60% will be suitable for, or want, endarterectomy.

Neuroimaging

CT shows an infarct relevant to the symptoms in about 25% of people who have had a TIA. MRI will show a lesion in 50%, including most of those who have symptoms lasting longer than an hour. A few will have an alternative diagnosis (tumours, multiple sclerosis), and very few will have small bleeds, and these may be saved further work-up and possible risks of carotid endarterectomy. Clinical uncertainty will indicate a scan in others (especially in determining vascular territory). If the symptoms last less than one hour, they can usually (but not definitely) be assumed to be ischaemic rather than bleeds.

Cardiological investigations

12-lead ECG to diagnose AF, evidence of ischaemic heart disease, and left ventricular hypertrophy. Follow this up with echocardiography if there is a history of cardiac disease, reason to suspect cardioembolism, or no other apparent cause in a younger patient (in which case bubble contrast or transoesophageal echocardiography is preferable).

Dealing with uncertainty

Correctly identifying TIA and its cause is difficult. Some doubt is inevitable. Overdiagnosis is as much a risk as missing true TIA:

- Get the process right. Careful history, perceptive examination, appropriate investigation, and explanation.
- Know the high-risk situations. Look carefully for evidence of stroke mimics, cardioembolism, tight carotid stenosis.
- A strong background in neurology can help identify difficult epilepsy or migraine, a background in general internal and geriatric medicine can help in diagnosis of syncope, cardiac disorders, and confusion.
- Seek second opinions and make specialist referrals if necessary.
- MRI (with DWI) can help (DWI positive cases have an increased risk of subsequent stroke), but MRI is not the whole answer to diagnostic uncertainty. You cannot rule out a TIA by investigation.

Give a balanced judgement and opinion. Don't diagnose TIA 'just in case'. Acknowledge the uncertainty, set out, in simple language, what is and is not known, and agree management with the patient (for example, whether to investigate further or start secondary prevention drugs). Lest there be doubt in future, it is sensible to put this in writing (e.g. by copying a GP letter to the patient).

Management of TIA

- All patients should be advised about general vascular prevention measures, including BP and cholesterol reduction, stopping smoking, and starting aspirin and dipyridamole.
- The time of greatest risk is the first couple of weeks after a TIA. Evidence suggests that secondary prevention should be started immediately—what components are most important is unclear. It is also unclear if BP should be reduced after measurement on a single occasion.
- Patients with a tight symptomatic stenosis should be offered endarterectomy within days (most of the potential benefit is lost after 2 weeks, virtually all of it after 3 months).
- Patients in AF should be counselled on the risks and benefits of anticoagulation (instead of aspirin/dipyridamole).
- Patients identified at very high risk still pose challenges on immediate intervention. Adding clopidogrel to aspirin for the 1st month is supported by sufficient evidence to make it reasonable, but this remains of uncertain benefit (see 📖 Boxes 10.5, p.243 and 10.21, p.274). There is little evidence to support the early use of dipyridamole. Early statins might have had some plaque stabilizing effect, but one small trial of early use was negative (see 📖 Box 10.5, p.243) and the main secondary prevention effect is seen after 12 months. However, they do little harm if started immediately.
- Management of comorbid diseases should be optimized, and an achievable drug regimen agreed.
- In cases of diagnostic uncertainty the decision for the clinician is whether the likelihood of TIA is sufficient to justify the burden of investigation, and possibly lifelong secondary prevention. It is reasonable to treat as a TIA if prognosis (judged by ABCD2 score or other evidence) is sufficiently worrying, and the duly informed patient is willing.

Preventing subarachnoid haemorrhage

- The key intervention (coiling or clipping the aneurysm) is designed to prevent rebleeding.
- With conservative management, after the first 3 months, rebleeding occurs at about 3% a year.
- Control of high BP and stopping smoking are epidemiologically sensible, if unproven by trial. In a large cohort, smoking more than doubled SAH risk, and each 10-mmHg decrease in systolic BP was associated with 31% reduced risk of SAH.
- People with two or more 1st- or 2nd-degree relatives with SAH are at increased risk (especially if there are two 1st-degree relatives, including a sibling). They may be considered for MRA screening, although there is no proven benefit from this approach.
- Intervening on asymptomatic aneurysms (detected during angiography after a bleed, or during imaging for another purpose, or because of screening of relatives) depends on the circumstances (Box 10.23). Risks are higher with older age (RR 1.06 per 1-year increase in age), aneurysm size (RR 1.05 per 1-mm increase), posterior circulation aneurysms, in women, and for aneurysms causing (non-SAH) symptoms (such as cranial nerve compression).

Box 10.23 Risk of rupture of asymptomatic aneurysms

- A cohort of 4060 patients with unruptured intracranial aneurysms was followed-up for up to 6 years. 1692 did not have aneurysm repair, 1917 had surgery, and 451 had endovascular treatment.

No history of subarachnoid haemorrhage (n=1077)

- 5-year risk of rupture for anterior circulation aneurysms (internal carotid, anterior communicating, anterior or middle cerebral arteries) was:
  - 0 for aneurysms <7mm.
  - 2.6% for aneurysms 7–12mm.
  - 14.5% for aneurysms 13–24mm.
  - 40% for aneurysms >25mm.
- 5-year risk of rupture for posterior circulation aneurysms (including posterior communicating arteries) was:
  - 2.5% for aneurysms <7mm.
  - 14.5% for aneurysms 7–12mm.
  - 18.4% for aneurysms 13–24mm.
  - 50% for aneurysms >25mm.
- Cavernous sinus carotid aneurysms were at less risk of rupture (0, 0, 3%, and 6% by size, over 5 years).
- The paradox is that small aneurysms are much more common than larger ones, so 60% of ruptured aneurysms are <5mm.

Patients with a history of SAH (from another aneurysm; n=615)

- Risk of rupture was similar to those without previous SAH apart from a 5-year risk of 1.5% (anterior circulation) and 3.4% (posterior circulation) for aneurysms <7mm.

Surgical and endovascular treatment

- 2.3% (surgery) and 3.1% (endovascular) died within a year, and 12.2% (surgery) and 9.5% (endovascular) had the combined poor outcome of death plus dependency or cognitive impairment a year after treatment.
- Age >50 years, aneurysms >12mm, posterior circulation aneurysms, non-rupture symptoms (e.g. cranial nerve palsy), and previous ischaemic stroke were associated with poor outcome after open surgery.
- Aneurysms >12mm, and posterior circulation aneurysms, but not age, were associated with poor outcome after coiling.

Conclusion

- Larger asymptomatic aneurysms are at high risk of rupture, but for most arteries <12mm, risks of surgery are as great or greater.

Lancet 2003; **362**:103–10.

Summary

1. Patients surviving a stroke are at high risk of another, and of other vascular events such as heart attacks. All should be considered for preventative interventions, but this should be tailored to the individual.
2. Use the principles of decision making discussed in 📖 Chapter 6, p.139 to help decide. Give the patient options or advice, rather than telling them what to do.
3. Unless contraindicated give antithrombotics (usually aspirin 75mg plus dipyridamole MR 200mg bd), or anticoagulant if that is specifically indicated.
4. Reduce BP as far as feasible without causing side effects.
5. Reduce cholesterol with a statin at high dose.
6. Screen for AF, and carotid stenosis in appropriate cases.
7. Advise smoking cessation, and refer to support services if necessary.
8. Advise weight loss, alcohol moderation, high fruit and vegetable diet, salt minimization, and regular exercise.
9. Make drug regimens feasible and as easy to take as possible. If in doubt about drug compliance, settle on an achievable regimen.
10. Rapid access neurovascular or TIA clinics are an option for investigation of transient neurological episodes, and should have access to carotid duplex scanning, and give comprehensive vascular preventative advice.
11. Asymptomatic intracranial aneurysms >12mm diameter justify prophylactic intervention.

Chapter 11

Outcomes and prognosis

Survival

This depends on (Table 11.1):
- Your perspective—community or hospital.
- The type of stroke, and indicators of its severity.
- When you are making your prediction. The longer after the stroke the better the chance of surviving the episode. Half of those who die in the 1st month, do so within the 1st week.
- The age and comorbidity of the patient.

For survivors, subsequent risks of dying are about twice those of the general population:
- 2.5% a year for those aged <65.
- 5% per year at ages 65–74.
- 10% per year for those aged >75.

Table 11.1 Survival after stroke

		1-month mortality	1-year mortality
Where	Community	15–25%	30–35%
	Hospital	20–30%	30–40%
Type	Haemorrhage	50%	60%
	TACI	40%	60%
	PACI	4%	16%
	LACI	2%	10%
	POCI	7%	20–30%
Features	Very severe (SSS <15)		62% (6 months)
	Severe (SSS 15–29)		34% (6 months)
	Moderate (SSS 30–44)		11% (6 months)
	Mild (SSS 45–58)		3% (6 months)

Survival after intracerebral bleeding is worse than after an infarct, and depends on location and severity. 1-year survival is:
- 49% for deep haemorrhage.
- 43% for lobar haemorrhage.
- 58% for cerebellar haemorrhage.
- 35% for brain stem haemorrhage.

Patients with initial GCS score <9 and haematoma volume ≥60mL have a mortality rate of 90% at 1 month, whereas patients with GCS ≥9 and a haematoma volume <30mL have a mortality of 17%. Risks are higher for those who bleed whilst on warfarin or aspirin. Mortality risk can be estimated using the ICH Score (Table 11.2).

Table 11.2 Prognosis of intracerebral haemorrhage based on the ICH Score (data from *Stroke* 2001; **32**:891–7)

		ICH score
Age	<80 years	0
	≥80 years	1
GCS at admission	13–15	0
	5–12	1
	3–4	2
Location	Supra-tentorial	0
	Infra-tentorial	1
Volume (ABC/2 method)	<30mL	0
	≥30mL	1
Intraventricular extension	No	0
	Yes	1

Score	30-day good outcome (%)	30-day mortality (%)
0	65	0
1	52	13
2	18	26
3	0	72
4	0	97
5+	0	100

ABC/2 method (for determining haemorrhage volume on CT scan) – multiply maximum haemorrhage length × width × number of slices on which it is visible × CT slice thickness and divide by 2.

Recurrence

TIA

The rate of recurrent TIA or stroke after a first TIA (or minor stroke) is:
- 10% within a week.
- 13% within a month.
- 18% within 3 months.

A third of these are fatal or disabling. After that annual rate of stroke is 5% and MI 2.5%. Early risk is 3-fold higher if the TIA or stroke is caused by large artery disease, and 5-fold lower if lacunar.

Risk of recurrence varies with:
- ABCD2 score (see 🕮 Box 10.22, p.276).
- Aetiological subtype.
- Presence of a visible infarct on MRI (38% risk of stroke at 90 days with a visible infarct on DWI; compared with 4% risk with none).

Cerebral infarction

Risk of fatal or disabling recurrence is:
- 5% in a month.
- 10–15% in the first year.
- 5% a year after that.

These data may be pessimistic, as they were collected before the more intensive preventative regimens used nowadays, which may halve the risk.

Recurrence rates are:
- Lower in younger people (<65 years) and people with milder strokes (perhaps 3–4% per year).
- Greater in older age (>80 years), continued smoking, higher BP and AF.

Aetiological inference or investigation can help determine risk of recurrence:
- Patients with partial anterior circulation or posterior circulation strokes, which are often embolic, have a high risk of recurrence (17–20%) over 1 year, concentrated in the first 6 months.
- Lacunar strokes recur at the rate of 9% over 1 year, and are more evenly spread over time.

Intracranial haemorrhage

After primary intracerebral haemorrhage (i.e. no identified cause) recurrent strokes occur at a rate of 7% per year. A third of these are bleeds, the rest infarcts. Risk is higher if the patient remains hypertensive. The rate of early recurrence (within 3 months) is about 1%.

Bleeds due to amyloid angiopathy (10% per year recurrence) and AVM (up to 30% per year recurrence) are especially prone to recurrence.

After SAH, risk of rebleeding from the culprit aneurysm without operation is very high (20% first day, 40% first month). Asymptomatic aneurysms have a 0–50% risk of bleeding over 5 years depending on their size and location (see 🕮 Box 10.13, p.259).

Neurological impairments and disabilities

What there is at the start, and how it changes, depends on:
- Which population you are studying. Hospital series tend to have worse strokes and more impairments.
- How carefully you look. Sophisticated testing for neglect and sensory impairments give initial prevalences up to 80%.
- When you look. Early on you will include features in those who recover or die very quickly.
- Comorbidity. Long follow-up of elderly populations is complicated by high death rates, recurrence, and comorbid events (like hip fractures).
- Mortality. The prevalence of severe paralysis decreases with time, because of very high mortality rather than recovery (Table 11.3).
- Intervention. Thrombolysis aims to avert established neurological damage, although 'cure' only occurs in about 1 in 10 thrombolysed cases.

For setting goals and giving information to individual patients, it is useful to know what the chances of recovery are for a given starting point, in particular the initial severity of the problem (Tables 11.4 and 11.5).

Table 11.3 Overall pattern of recovery of arm and leg weakness in a community stroke register, South London Stroke Register (data courtesy of Dr Enas Lawrence)

	Initial	3 months	1 year	2 years
Sample	1259	1259	943	295
Died	18%	37%	44%	51%
Lost	0	4%	4%	8%
Recurrence	0	3%	7%	8%
Arm				
No weakness	15%	23%	25%	22%
Mild	27%	19%	15%	10%
Moderate	10%	7%	6%	4%
Severe	20%	7%	4%	5%
Leg				
No weakness	18%	24%	28%	24%
Mild	26%	19%	13%	8%
Moderate	12%	8%	7%	5%
Severe	14%	5%	4%	4%

Table 11.4 Initial incidence and recovery from various neurological impairments

Impairment	Initially affected	Recovery and residual impairment
Arm and leg motor function	75%	80% show some recovery. Most within 3–6 weeks. Little improvement after 3 months, but some individuals improve up to a year. Flaccidity and initial severe weakness have poorer prognosis
Hemianopia	25%	Recovers quickly if at all, mostly within 10 days. Little recovery after 28 days. 80% of complete hemianopias, and 30% of partial field losses persist (50% and 10% respectively die)
Visual and sensory inattention	20% each	Perhaps half recover
Sensory loss	30%	Perhaps half recover
Aphasia	25%	Initial severe aphasia, 50% survivors remain moderately or severely affected
		Initial moderate aphasia, 15% of survivors persist no better or worse
		Initial mild aphasia, 9% have persisting problems. Little recovery after 10 weeks
Dysarthria	25%	Generally recovers
Cognition	25%	Initially difficult to estimate due to drowsiness or aphasia. Some recovery may occur over 6–12 months.10–20% have persisting problems
Urinary incontinence	50%	A third of initially-incontinent patients recover within 4 weeks. 20% of 6-month survivors are incontinent
Faecal incontinence	30%	10% of 6-month survivors are incontinent
Walking (any assistance)	60%	64% survivors independent, 14% with assistance, 22% remain unable to walk at 6 months. Some further recovery possible between 6–12 months

- Useful function in the arm is unlikely if there is no return in grip after a month.
- If there is some return of arm muscle activity by a month, some large joint movement is likely to recover.
- Hand function recovers last and least.
- Arms and legs recover at about the same speed and to approximately the same extent (although the leg is slightly less often severely affected).

Table 11.5 Recovery according to initial level of function (Copenhagen Stroke Study)

Function	Initial severity	Recovery at 6 months
Arms	Mild–moderate weakness	80% good function, 20% no recovery (10% die)
	Severe weakness	17% of survivors recover good function, another 17% recover partially (40% die)
Legs	Complete paralysis	12% of survivors regain independent walking, 12% walk with assistance (56% die)
	Moderate–severe weakness (without complete paralysis)	40% of survivors regain independent walking, 20% walk with assistance (30% die)
	Mild weakness	80% of survivors regain independent walking, 10% walk with assistance (10% die)
Walking	Unable	22% of survivors eventually walk independently, 22% walk with assistance (40% die)
	With assistance	60% of survivors eventually get independent, 35% walk with assistance (5% die)
Aphasia	Mild	Reach a plateau within 2 weeks. Half recover completely, most of the rest remain mildly affected (20% die)
	Moderate	Reach a plateau within 6 weeks. Half of survivors recover completely, another 40% remain mildly affected (30% die)
	Severe	Reach a plateau within 10 weeks. A quarter of survivors recover completely, another quarter remain mildly affected. (70% die)

Independence

- Half of survivors are independent in basic ADL after 6 months (but only 20% for those suffering an intracerebral bleed).
- By 1 year 60% of survivors are independent, largely because the most disabled have died, rather than real recovery. Another 20% are no more than mildly disabled.
- 20% of survivors require institutional care 1 year after their stroke.
- Prognosis for independence at 1 year varies by stroke subtype:
  - TACI 4% overall (10% of survivors).
  - PACI 60% overall (70% of survivors).
  - LACI 60% overall (67% of survivors).
  - POCI 60% overall (75% of survivors).
- Prognosis for independence at 1 year varies by initial neurological severity (SSS score):
  - Very severe (SSS <15):   4%
  - Severe (SSS 15–29):   13%
  - Moderate (SSS 30–44):   37%
  - Mild (SSS 45–58):   68%.

Discharge

- Discharge prospects vary with initial stroke severity (Table 11.6).
- One-third of survivors of severe strokes are discharged home with no more than mild disability.

Table 11.6 Discharge destination according to initial severity (Copenhagen Stroke Study)

	Died	Own home	Nursing home
Very severe (SSS <15)	62%	23%	14%
Severe (SSS 15–29)	34%	34%	32%
Moderate (SSS 30–44)	11%	75%	14%
Mild (SSS 45–58)	3%	93%	4%

Outcome of subarachnoid haemorrhage

- 25% die within 24h.
- 50% die within 3 months.

Mortality from SAH, and dependency among the survivors, are quite high, but vary with:

- The patient's age.
- Level of consciousness at onset (Table 11.7).
- Angiographic findings (perimesencephalic better than aneurysmal; anterior better than posterior circulation).
- CT findings (perimesencephalic distribution, amount of blood, intra-ventricular blood).
- Focal neurological signs.

The majority of 'good grade' patients will make a good recovery. Amongst coiled or clipped patients in the ISAT trial, 5-year mortality was 11–14%, and 83% of survivors were functionally independent (see 📖 Box 4.2, p.103). However, a few initially comatose patients will also recover well.

Table 11.7 Overall outcomes 6 months after SAH (data from *Journal of Neurosurgery* 1990; 73:18–36)

Level of consciousness on admission	Mortality (%)	Good recovery (%)
Alert	13%	74%
Drowsy	28%	54%
Stuperose	44%	30%
Comatose	72%	11%

Summary

1. Overall, 1-month mortality after a stroke is 20–30% and 1-year mortality 30–40%.
2. However, survival is very variable depending on age, type of stroke, and indicators of severity. Prognosis for some is very much better.
3. Stroke recurrence is 10% in the first year, 5% a year after that.
4. Survivors of stroke recover to some extent. 4% of patients with very severe strokes recover to independence, whereas 70% of mild strokes do. The majority will regain walking, independently or with assistance.
5. Overall 30–40% of patients (70% of survivors) are left with no more than mild limb weakness. There is little neurological recovery after 3 months, although functional recovery continues longer, especially for the most severely affected.
6. Between 20% (initially very severe) and 90% (initially mild) will achieve discharge home.
7. About half of SAH patients die, but most of the remainder make a good functional recovery.

Chapter 12

Longer-term problems and their management

Introduction

Hospital management of stroke represents the start not the end of the story for many patients and their families. Services must identify and address their longer-term needs as well.

Many report a feeling of abandonment after leaving hospital. Intensive rehabilitation and hospital discharge processes give way to a new set of problems with little specialist support. Problems persist for many years, and health professionals may appear negative and unhelpful.

The hospital practitioner can anticipate problems, should know what follow-on rehabilitation or support services are available, may be able to help prepare the patient and carers for what is to come, and should hand over thoroughly to community services.

Some issues—such as mobility, continence, and cognitive problems, spasticity, shoulder pain, or low mood—may persist from earlier, but may evolve, or change with circumstances.

Other problems emerge later, some relating to resettlement and readjustment. Issues include return to work, driving, re-establishing interests, hobbies, social life, and social or civic participation.

Services are criticized by patients and carers for limiting their goals to physical function, achieving independence in basic ADL, and secondary prevention. However, precisely which additional aspects to target, and how to help, have been difficult to define. Patients and carers may be reluctant to ask for help, so a proactive approach is needed.

Current UK guidelines are vague, calling for:
• Psychosocial support.
• Information.
• Driving advice.
• A 6-month reassessment.
• A named service contact.

Expertise on what to do can be found in community rehabilitation services, where they exist, and by drawing on the experience of services for other chronic neurological conditions.

What problems?

Box 12.1 Longer-term problems after a stroke

Domains	Subdomains
Social and emotional	Social
	Emotional
	Attitude to recovery
	Relationships and self-perception
Services	Social
	Health
Hospital discharge	Preparation for living at home
	Abandonment
Communication	Written
	Verbal
Hospital experience	Therapy
	Critical events

British Journal of General Practice 2003; **53**:803–7.

Patients' problems

The biggest problem area is 'social and emotional'.

Different *emotional* consequences of stroke are described in up to 60% of cases. An emotion is a mental and physiological state associated with feelings, thoughts, and behaviours, such as vulnerability, lack of confidence, anxiety, depression, or anger. Emotions are subjective, and may be associated with personality. Depression and anxiety figure highly amongst complaints in the years after a stroke.

Social consequences include:
● 30% unable to go to the shops.
● 30% feel isolated.
● Only 20% of drivers return to driving.
● Only 10–20% of those previously employed return to work.

Patients may feel incapable of doing the activities that formed the basis of their previous social world, and become excluded from it, yet lack the abilities, skills, or resources to build a new one.

There are numerous impediments to social reintegration, including fatigue, embarrassment, fear, speech and cognitive problems, and physical and environmental obstacles. Self-esteem problems include feelings of uncertainty, and loss of identity and independence. Personal relationships can be strained because of forced changes in role, overprotective behaviour by carers, and attempts to maintain a façade of normality.

Both patients and carers continue to reflect on *negative hospital and discharge experiences,* even many months later. A third report dissatisfaction with discharge preparation. Lack of communication, especially written information, is commonly reported.

Service deficiencies, include both health and social care, with instances of broken promises of help, delays, unreliable or inflexible home care, and difficulty in accessing adaptations, equipment, and financial disability benefits. Half of patients in the UK see their GP within 6 weeks of discharge and three-quarters within a year, but a third feel dissatisfied with medical care. Patients would prefer long-term specialist medical follow-up.

Patients and carers frequently perceived a need for *further rehabilitation* after discharge from hospital. Patients are frustrated by what is provided, with inappropriate goal setting, and continued concentration on physical function. Health professionals are described as being negative about the prospects for recovery beyond 6 months from stroke onset, reflecting an undue concentration on neurological impairment at the expense of new learning, compensation and adaptation, and addressing psychological barriers to function and reintegration.

Two-thirds of patients are dissatisfied with the support that they receive from *Social Services.*

Carer problems

Looking after a disabled person has physical, psychological, and social consequences for the carer (see Box 12.2). Supporting carers is necessary:
- To sustain the health of the carer.
- To sustain support for the patient, which would otherwise reduce choice, possibly requiring increased professional support, or care home placement.

Three-quarters of carers feel ill-prepared for their role. They report emotional distress, problems coping, anxiety, depression, and tiredness. Half report physical ill-health.

Two-thirds report limitation in social activities, 20% isolation. One-third perceive deterioration in their relationship with the patient, and a third sexual difficulties.

A number of different types of stress have been identified amongst carers, including:
- Identity: the problems of changing from a spouse or child, into a carer.
- Self-esteem: may be damaged by a caring role.
- Bereavement: individuals typically grieve the loss of the person prior to their stroke, and a future they had been looking forward to. Retirement plans rarely include looking after an incapacitated spouse and people may become angry about the injustice of what they have lost.

Factors making caring more stressful include:
- The carer living with care recipient.
- Incontinence, especially faecal.
- Interrupted sleep.
- Inability to communicate.
- Loss of companionship and reciprocity.
- Social life being limited.
- Poor quality of prior relationship.
- Difficulty getting away on holiday.
- Feeling that one has been pressured into caring.
- Cultural pressures.

Coping depends on:
- Physical resources: material and financial.
- Social resources: family and social networks.
- Psychological resources: the carer's personality and coping mechanisms.
- Carers' perception of disability and disturbed behaviour.

Those with more 'intrinsic motivators', such as admiration, or a strong prior relationship, experienced lower levels of stress. Carer satisfaction comes from continued reciprocity and mutual affection, companionship, job satisfaction, and fulfilment of sense of duty.

Men and women can differ in their response to social support. Men tend to be grateful for any input from domiciliary services and are relieved of some of their stress. Women feel more guilty about needing to rely on outside help, which may make them feel inadequate.

Box 12.2 Who is a carer?

'Someone who looks after a partner, relative or friend, because of illness, disability, frailty, or the effects of old age.'

An alternative definition captures the idea of burden imposed by caring responsibilities: 'Someone whose life is restricted by the need to be responsible for the care of someone who is mentally ill, mentally handicapped, physically disabled or whose health is impaired by sickness or old age' (Pitkeathley J, *It's my Duty, Isn't it?* London: Souvenir Press, 1989).

The term carer (or caregiver) is loose and variably-defined. Organizations representing unpaid carers (sometimes called 'informal carers') seek to draw a distinction from paid ('statutory' or 'professional') carers.

Some carers provide direct physical care, sometimes very intensive and intimate, others provide intermittent help with more difficult tasks (bills, shopping, household maintenance), others may provide emotional support, advocacy, oversight, or help arranging support.

Difficult questions include:
- Who decides you are a carer and when do you cease to be a carer?
- What is normal 'helping' (e.g. sharing jobs within a family) and what is special 'caring'?
- Are you still a carer if your relative is placed in residential or nursing care?
- How long after the death of a relative do you cease to be a carer?
- Are you legally defined as a carer by health and social services? (In the UK, carers are entitled to an assessment of their own needs, and may be paid benefits depending on the amount of time spent caring and the entitlement to benefits of the person receiving care).

Adjustment, psychological and emotional recovery

Adjustment is the psychological process of coming to terms with a new reality, the setting of new goals and ambitions, and reintegration to social and civic life. Many of the 'social and emotional' problems described after stroke represent a failure to readjust. Patients may be angry and resentful about being disabled. Inpatient rehabilitation is necessarily optimistic, both because of uncertainty about prognosis early after stroke, but also to bolster morale and engagement. The change of direction from 'expectation of recovery' to 'planning to cope with disability' can be hard.

The loss of optimistic outlook and professional guidance can cause the sense of abandonment. Loss of function is blamed on inadequate therapy, or critical incidents (e.g. delay in seeking help, starting therapy, or feeding, or a fall). General dissatisfaction becomes 'lack of information'.

Four types of interventions have been tried:
- Education: about stroke, its effects, prevention, and about what different services are available and how to access them.
- Peer support (e.g. via voluntary or carers' organizations).
- Therapy: formal psychological therapy following a specific model, or less structured 'emotional support' from nurses, community therapists, or specially employed family support workers. These may be based on problem-solving or stress-coping theories. One problem is that calls for 'emotional' or 'psychosocial' support are vague, and health professionals with a background in physical health are unaware of psychological approaches and how to access them.
- Practical support: sometimes the 'emotional' difficulty is rooted in problems surrounding ADL, behaviour, availability of personal care support services or specialized equipment.

These interventions are not mutually exclusive, and multiple approaches are usually appropriate, resulting in complex packages of care:
- Support workers or nurses. Promoting adjustment is central to their role. They can respond flexibly to different, and unpredictable, needs. Intervention centres on identifying problems, providing information, sympathetic listening, reassurance, counselling, advocacy, and coordinating access to community and hospital services.
- Multidisciplinary community rehabilitation and support services. In theory, they should be well placed to address many longer-term problems, including restorative or adaptive rehabilitation of function in the home or local environment, involvement of family and carers, supply of equipment, and ensuring the establishment of social care services. They can have more overt readjustment roles as well. For example, one function of 'leisure occupational therapy' is to identify the valued aspect of an activity and either redirect or reset it. Someone who enjoyed the competitive side of sport, for example, might rediscover competitive chess. Mental health nurses or clinical psychologists can engage in more formal counselling or cognitive behavioural therapies.

- Medical (or nursing) review at 6 months (mandated in the UK by national guidelines), screening for outstanding problems, giving advice and information, and referral back to therapy or other services where an unmet need is identified. Much of the 'intervention' here is advice, with occasional referral back to rehabilitation therapies or specialized services such as spasticity management.
- Patient and carer education and training programmes: skills are imparted to promote recovery and enable self-maintenance, e.g. gait pattern, falls prevention, protection of a hemiplegic shoulder or a spastic limb. Carers can have a major influence, helpful or otherwise. On the one hand they can be supportive and partners in change. On the other they can be overprotective or foster dependency, depriving the person of independence or 'agency' (the ability to make choices). Education programmes aim to help patients and carers adjust to stroke by increasing their knowledge about stroke, recovery, rehabilitation, and availability of services. Strategies which actively involve patient and carers have a greater effect on patient anxiety and depression than passive strategies (such as giving leaflets). Specifically training carers in basic therapy and nursing tasks can improve both patients' and carers' psychological health (see 📖 Box 8.9, p.215).

None of these approaches appears to have a major impact on function. All increase satisfaction, knowledge about stroke, and improve carer (and sometimes patient) psychological well-being. There is a clear need for an access point back to specialist services, when problems evolve or new ones develop—such as worsening spasticity or shoulder pain. Resource-limited services can be reluctant to provide such open-ended support.

Negotiation of goals is important. The difference between ambitious and unrealistic can be subtle. The reacquisition of abilities is one approach to achieving goals, but may prove impossible. Suggesting this can be a point of conflict between patients, carers, and rehabilitation professionals. Where a goal appears to be unrealistic, services can offer periods of assessment (of problems and response to therapy), and setting of intermediate goals (something that will have to be achieved first if the ambitious longer-term goal is to be met).

Some effects of intervention are counterintuitive. Many carers feel the need for a break, but out-of-home respite care (i.e. in a care home) may not alleviate carer's stress, if it causes resentment in the care recipient. In-home respite (sitting services) and day care tend to reduce stress more.

Functional issues

Many stroke survivors underperform once home. They do not go back to doing things that they could do, often lacking confidence, or fearing falls or stroke recurrence. Adapting to the out-of-hospital environment provides new challenges—your own particular stairs have to be climbed, and your own kitchen used for meal preparation, whilst a range of potential new goals becomes relevant, such as outdoor mobility, or return to work. Community rehabilitation services can be effective here, e.g. accompanied journeys by taxi or bus, or to the shops, can demonstrate what is possible and increase confidence.

Occupation and activity needs vary, depending on type of impairment (e.g. aphasia) or severity. The voluntary sector and local social services are the main providers of clubs, groups, and day centres. These are a focus for providing information and support, and reducing isolation, as well as a change of routine and environment.

Specialized organizations may advise on provision or opportunities for those with disabilities, such as fishing or gardening. The problem is often knowing where to look—the internet is useful, as are charities directories, and informal contacts ('the grapevine').

Maintenance of ability is important. Over time people may deteriorate, through stroke recurrence or comorbid medical problems, deconditioning, or the acquisition of bad habits. Periodic 'maintenance therapy' can help (e.g., in improving walking speed), although how much, and how often is not well defined.

How this works in practice depends on the healthcare system. Ongoing therapy can be difficult to access unless there is a catastrophe or crisis. It is easy to argue that periodic routine medical follow-up has little to offer in practical terms, but it can provide a route back to therapy services when a need does become apparent.

Fatigue

Many stroke survivors describe a feeling of continual exhaustion. Fatigue is an enhanced perception of effort and limited endurance for sustained physical and mental activity.

Aetiology is poorly understood, but may include depression, fear, loss of motivation, pain, sleep disturbance, deconditioning, hormonal (hypothalamo–pituitary–adrenal axis) or specific neurological damage.

Poststroke fatigue occurs in around 50% of patients, including 30% of those who have had a minor stroke. Some patients, having made an apparently excellent neurological recovery complain bitterly about fatigue. Amongst inpatients, therapists frequently report therapy being limited by fatigue. In the longer term, it is a major barrier to return to normal activities, including work.

Fatigue is reported in many long-term neurological and non-neurological diseases, including multiple sclerosis, cancer, rheumatoid arthritis, and fibromyalgia, as well as up to 20% of the general population. It can last more than a year after the event, and characteristically has a different quality from usual fatigue, with a poor response to rest.

What to do:
- Ask about it routinely.
- Assess for depression.
- Ask about sleep.
- Consider reversible causes (e.g. anaemia, hypothyroidism, infection).
- Assess pain and spasticity.
- Note overweight, alcohol use, and sleep apnoea syndrome.
- Review drugs (e.g. beta-blockers, other antihypertensives, statins, sedatives, antipsychotics and antidepressants).

There is no proven beneficial treatment. On average, people who have had a stroke are only half as fit as age-matched controls (measured by peak oxygen consumption), despite having increased energy demands during common activities. This can manifest as exercise intolerance. Progressive, graded aerobic and strength exercise training, or, if available, cognitive behavioural therapy, are most likely to help. A practical hint is to 'keep trying things', with the aim of keeping the patient active and engaged allowing spontaneous recovery to occur without the complications of severe deconditioning, detachment, and increasing social isolation.

'Pacing' (limiting activity to prevent exhaustion) is a popular strategy amongst suffers of fatiguing conditions, and whilst there are clearly limits on what a fatigued person can achieve, emphasizing this is as likely to perpetuate the problem as alleviate it. Advice on exercise should be that it is regularity rather than intensity that is important. Cognitive strategies (distraction, prioritization) can also help.

Low-dose tricyclic antidepressants (amitriptyline, trazodone) or antiepileptic drugs (gabapentin, valproate) may be tried (but often make matters worse). Amantadine is used for fatigue in multiple sclerosis, modafinil in some other conditions. There is little experience in stroke.

Spasticity

Limbs with high tone need constantly looking after, and if neglected will inevitably suffer complications. These include loss of range of movement (contracture or flexion deformity at the hand or elbow; ankle plantar-flexion), leading to pain, hand hygiene problems, and loss of function. Problems are most likely in people with severe paralysis. However, unlike progressive neurological conditions, there is potential to stabilize a vulnerable limb after a stroke.

In the early phase after stroke, during the first month or so, specialist multidisciplinary management is usually successful. It is after discharge, when careful regular supervision by therapists and nurses ceases, that problems arise. Some form of follow-up is therefore required, by a knowledgeable physician, nurse, or physiotherapist. Developing problems must be addressed early, before they become irreversible.

Patients (or carers, or care home staff) should be taught the importance of:
• Passive stretching at least twice a day.
• Suitable posture (sitting up, arm supported) in appropriate seating or wheelchair.
• Use of splints (applied 2–4h, twice a day, and/or overnight if possible).
• Avoidance of aggravators or 'nociceptive stimuli'—pain, constipation, blocked catheters, pressure sores.
• Early referral if problems are worsening.

Early intervention makes management easier. Most places should have access to a specialist spasticity clinic, managed by neurorehabilitationists, neurologists or stroke physicians. Reassessment requires involvement of doctor, physiotherapist, occupational therapist, and orthotist.

Management involves relieving exacerbating factors, injection of botulinum toxin to relieve overactive muscles, then stretching and splinting, or serial casting (changing casts progressively to increase range of joint movement).

Treating exacerbating factors includes dealing with a painful shoulder, itself difficult and contentious. However, a suprascapular nerve block can be useful in conjunction with other measures. The nerve block causes numbness in the shoulder for about a week, to enable physiotherapists to work with the patient. The nerve block can be repeated.

Half will need botulinum toxin injection, and about 25% repeated injection. However, botulinum toxin alone is not a solution. It needs to be used as part of multidisciplinary management and follow-up.

Problems predominate with arm flexors and leg extensors.

In the lower limb, the most common problem is ankle plantar flexion and inversion (gastrocnemius, soleus, tibialis posterior). Hip adductors and hamstrings can be a problem especially if the patient does not walk. Extensor hallucis longus overactivity (striate toe) can produce pain on walking.

In the upper limb, problems occur with hand flexors (flexor digitorum superficialis and profundus, flexor pollicis longus), wrist flexors (flexor carpi ulnaris and radialis), pronation (pronator teres), elbow flexion (biceps, brachioradialis, brachialis), shoulder abduction (pectoralis major), and internal rotation (subscapularis and teres major).

Electromyography or nerve stimulation can be used to identify the most overactive muscles. These can then be injected with botulinum toxin. This starts to become effective within a few days to a week, with maximum effect at 2 weeks and duration of action about 12 weeks. 2 weeks after injection the patient should be reassessed for response, for more physiotherapy and resplinting. A second dose may be required. Effect should be documented using an appropriate before and after measure (range of movement, photograph, pain visual analogue scale, Ashworth scale, patient or carer functional rating scale). Problems include local effects (bruising or pain), diffusion to other muscles (causing unintended weakness) and, very rarely, dysphagia, generalized weakness or botulism.

Oral muscle relaxing agents (baclofen, tizanidine, dantrolene, diazepam) are rarely useful.

A related problem is that of 'associated reactions'. This is an involuntary movement of part of the body on the affected side in response to effort at another body site. This can be troublesome functionally (e.g. 'storking'— involuntary flexion of hip and knee during standing). It is usually associated with increased tone. Both physiotherapy and injected botulinum toxin can help.

In severe cases of contracture, often indicating poor previous management, surgical tendon release can be considered.

Aphasia

People with aphasia describe changes in communication over some years after a stroke. Very severe early aphasics sometimes 'come out of a fog' 6 months (or more) later—they may start to respond to therapy for the first time. This, and the long-term challenges of living with aphasia, make it important to have ongoing access to expert help from a speech and language therapist.

An approach assessing impairments, functional problems, and context is used. Management of communication problems is based on goals agreed with the patient. Ask the patient what communication needs and goals they have. Supported conversation resources (pictures, words, symbols) are available to facilitate this discussion. If goals are thought to be unrealistic, either a time-limited period of assessment, or work on an agreed intermediate goal, are instituted.

The approach depends on the problem. However, four main strategies are employed:

- *Work to improve impairments.* A thorough neuropsychologically-based assessment determines the location of the language block. This can still help beyond 6 months after stroke onset, when spontaneous recovery is complete. Work to overcome problems requires motivation and intensive therapy, including the use of computer programs. Opportunities to improve impairments should not be missed or overlooked, but only rarely will this produce a major benefit in terms of functional communication.
- *Compensation.* Various approaches are employed. Circumlocution is the device of thinking or talking round the meaning of a word that cannot be found. Cueing, by the patient or by the conversation partner, can also help. There are various methods: 'how do you spell it?', 'what is the first letter?' (graphemic), saying the first sound (phonological), visualization. Alternative communication strategies such as writing (or partial writing, e.g. writing the first letter of a word), use of communication books, pictures, or other preprepared resources can be used. Therapy aims to promote spontaneous (i.e. unprompted) use of compensation strategies.
- *Promoting adjustment.* The social and emotional effects of aphasia are profound. Sometimes therapy is best delayed beyond the acute phase when the emotional impact is too intense to allow progress. This also avoids the experience of early speech therapy being dominated by the experience of failure. A counselling approach is used, listening and reflecting, identifying and articulating problems, and exploring potential solutions. This alone can be helpful even in the absence of any 'action'. Aphasia can also put strains on relationships, and relationship counselling is important. People with aphasia often cannot access regular counselling services, making the role of the speech therapist all the more important. Some subspecialized speech therapists are dual trained in counselling.
- *Supporting families and carers.* A lot involves teaching and information, and coaching in supported conversation. Problems can arise with

unwanted completion of sentences, and failure to allow turn-taking. Video analysis may be used to highlight this. Someone with a fluent aphasia may not realize that they have a problem. Carers also have emotional and support needs.

Occupation and activity can be restricted in aphasia. Films or television programmes can be too difficult to follow (to make them interesting they are often fast moving, with complex story lines, and partial or unstated information). People with aphasia often miss the ability to read. Some non-linguistic activities such as gardening are popular. Most shopping can be done without speaking (using a credit card PIN number can be practised). Return to work may be possible, but is difficult if aphasia is severe. If not, voluntary work is an alternative, and the client needs advice on what is possible and suitable. Aphasia per se is not a bar to driving (although associated cognitive and physical impairments may be).

Group work (under banners such as 'total communication groups' and 'supported conversation groups') plays an important part in ongoing therapy, and contribute to different objectives. As well as providing peer support, and support for family members, groups can help with learning compensation strategies and adjustment, and maintaining social skills which can quickly become neglected with a communication impairment.

Late reassessment depends on an assessment of functional communication, problems manifest, and goals identified. The therapist looks for evidence of spontaneous use of compensation. Problems can arise when inappropriate compensation strategies are used (e.g. a relative finishing sentences or taking over speech).

Driving

(See ✌ http://www.dvla.gov.uk; medical rules)

In the UK, driving is permitted if safe, 1 month after the stroke (or a TIA). The final decision on granting a licence lies with the Driver and Vehicle Licensing Agency (DVLA), who may take advice from medical staff involved. The driver's insurer must also be informed, or the insurance may become invalid.

- Severe disability precluding driving should be obvious to all concerned, but identifying cognitive disabilities making driving unsafe may be more difficult, especially where insight is lacking.
- A hemianopia precludes driving.
- Epilepsy regulations hold (for car drivers, a fit within the first 24h of a stroke can be discounted; otherwise no driving for a year after a fit, or whilst withdrawing antiepileptic drugs, or for 6 months after complete discontinuation of drugs).
- Following frequent TIAs, there must be 3 months free of attacks.
- Heavy Goods Vehicle (HGV) and Public Service (PSV) licences can be restored after at least 12 months, if a full and complete recovery from stroke or TIA has been made.
- Specialist neurological occupational therapists may be able to do a paper and pencil screening assessment (the Stroke Driver's Screening Assessment) to identify those likely to have driving problems.
- A simulator or test track assessment at a specialist mobility centre may be required (for a fee). These centres can also advise on vehicle adaptation and offer retraining, e.g. to rebuild confidence.

Exercise, physical activity, and sex

- Graded exercise is encouraged where physically possible, without restriction, not least in order to maintain physical function and as part of secondary prevention.
- Another stroke is unlikely during sex. Staff should make it clear that discussion of sex is legitimate, and someone willing to talk about it identified in advance of the question arising. Sexual problems may reflect fear of another stroke, communication problems, relationship problems, depression, the effects of physical disability or incontinence, or impotence. Barriers caused by physical disabilities might be helped by trying new positions or non-penetrative love-making. Suggest (or refer on to) relationship counsellors if necessary, including specialists for people with disabilities (e.g. in the UK, Relate and Outsiders).
- Drugs can cause lack of libido and impotence (including antihypertensives and antidepressants). Impotence may also be caused by comorbid diseases, such as diabetes and peripheral vascular disease.
- Standard management of erectile dysfunction can be used for patients with stroke, including phosphodiesterase inhibitors (if not on nitrates), alprostidil urethral suppositories (MUSE), or mechanical devices.

Holidays

Issues include physical capability of travelling, enjoyment whilst away, and risk of recurrence.

Anyone able to transfer between a car and a wheelchair should be able to travel most places, although long journeys can be stressful, and consideration must be given to toileting en route. Access to public toilets for a carer of the opposite sex is a problem. The physical environment in some places may not be as well adapted for people with disabilities as it is at home, including steps and stairs.

Whether to take this on is a matter of personal choice, but people welcome advice from professionals, and should be helped to anticipate potential practical problems. If someone does not want to contemplate the risk of getting ill abroad, clearly they should not travel. However, the risks of recurrence are relatively low, after the first few months at least, and most holiday destinations have good access to healthcare if needed.

Adequate travel and health insurance is vital—and pre-existing health conditions must be declared.

Requests to certify that someone is unfit for travel for insurance purposes can be difficult to manage, as desire to travel after a serious illness is so subjective.

Flying is allowed 3 days after a stroke so long as the person is stable or improving, but the airline should be informed in advance if the stroke was recent or disabling (see 🖱 http://www.britishairways.com; information; health and well-being).

Child care, adult caregiver skills

Stroke survivors can do what is possible and safe. Professional staff will often be faced with being asked for advice in areas where they feel they have no specific training. Know your limits, but explore the problems, discuss them at multidisciplinary meetings, and think broadly and laterally in suggesting solutions.

Return to work

Vocational rehabilitation is 'the process in which those disadvantaged by illness or disability are enabled to access, maintain, or return to employment, or other useful occupation'. 15% of stroke patients are in paid employment at the time of their stroke. Only 20% return to work (Table 12.1). This is unfamiliar territory for many health professionals.

Table 12.1 Survey of younger stroke survivors' experiences of return to work (data from *Getting back to work after stroke*; Stroke Association, London, 2006)

Want to return to work		75%
Of whom ...	did not feel fit enough to work	48%
Not working 1 year after stroke		83%
Of whom ...	forced to retire by employer	19%
	can't meet work expectations	30%
	can't drive/use public transport	31%
	afraid of losing disability benefits	32%
	did not feel fit enough to work	61%
	no longer feel able to do previous job	62%

Evidence suggests that work is good for you. Benefits include:
• More income and less dependence on state benefits.
• Enhanced sense of purpose and self-worth.
• A structured daily routine.
• Social contact.
• Better mood and mental health.
• Better physical health.

Enabling people with disabilities to return to work has become a major policy goal, with considerable resources and expertise available to help. This means access to vocational assessment, rehabilitation, and ongoing support to enable people with disabilities to find, regain, or remain in work, or other occupational and educational opportunities. Return to work rates of 50–70% may be possible. For someone who wants to return to work, eventually some form of employment can usually be found, even if they are moderately disabled.

Health and non-health factors both have a bearing on chances of success:
• The nature and severity of the health problem.
• Prior education and skills (those with better education and skills are more successful).
• Nature of the work (non-manual occupations are more successful).
• Length of time off work.
• General employment and unemployment rates.
• Attitudes to people with disabilities working.

If those who want to return to work do not receive proper advice, they may:

- Not realize the possibility of returning to work or alternative occupation.
- Return too soon, or resume full duties too quickly, and fail (affecting perhaps 20% of people who try).

Problems with fine motor skills, communication, cognition, working speed, concentration, and organizational abilities may limit capacity to work in the competitive job market. These 'hidden disabilities' are often missed, or left unaddressed by the time someone leaves hospital. Emotional vulnerability may reduce capacity to cope with pressure or responsibility, irritability, or overt expressions of frustration may cause difficulties in relationships with colleagues, and disinhibited or aggressive behaviour is rarely tolerated in the workplace. Lack of insight limits capacity to self-monitor and self-manage problems.

Fatigue and cognitive and executive problems often result in failure. Patients may feel constrained to go back to work for financial reasons or through fear of losing their job. They may not tell their employer or colleagues about their stroke, but get noticed as things go wrong, then give up or get dismissed. After a moderate or severe stroke physical disabilities preclude early return to work. Whilst waiting for rehabilitation or improvement, contact with the employer is lost, and return to the previous job may become impossible simply through lack of information or communication.

In general, the longer someone is off work, the lower the chance of successfully returning to work. However, after a moderately disabling stroke, return to work before 6 months has passed can be unwise. This usually coincides with the allowance for sick leave, so is not too much of a problem for employers.

Ideally, intervention should start early. We should at least ask if someone was working, and if they want to try to return. If someone is a hospital inpatient or significantly disabled, the question of working arises through the need for sickness certification. Someone, on the brink of retirement, however, may choose to retire early instead.

After minor non-disabling stroke or TIA issues may also arise. Problems include driving restrictions (getting to work, work-related driving), or where safety risks may be difficult to quantify (e.g. crane or machinery operators).

Try to keep all options open. Avoid making an early decision to stop working—wait at least 6 months poststroke. 'It's too early to tell' is a reasonable position. But keep the issue live. Anticipate likely problems. Encourage early contact with the employer, and complete openness and honesty—but seek the patient's consent if staff contact the employer. Information disclosed to an employer or occupational health should be discussed and agreed in advance.

People need support, guidance, or rehabilitation for:
- Job retention—returning to your old job.
- Retraining—identifying and preparing for alternative work.
- Maintaining re-employment—successfully staying in employment.
- Planning withdrawal from work, conserving pension and other rights (retiring on health grounds).
- Seeking alternative occupation or education opportunities (e.g. volunteering or attendance at a sheltered workshop).

The process comprises:
- Assess the person (vocational assessment): physical, cognitive, insight, behavioural problems, previous employment, skills and qualifications, previous return to work efforts, ambitions, and attitudes.
- Assess the job, and compare abilities with job demands (job analysis). Identify specific risks or restrictions, and how physical and cognitive deficits might manifest.
- Problem solve. Assess if work modification is possible, if parts of work can be reassigned to another employee, or reallocation to alternative work is required.
- Decide if specific vocational rehabilitation, or other work preparation, is required.
- Decide if specific external support (e.g. a support worker, equipment, or travel assistance is needed).
- Follow-up for new or emerging problems.

Advice should be sought from various sources or stakeholders:
- Employer.
- Patient.
- Occupational health practitioners, who provide advice to employee and employer about the prospects for and the process of return to work and the management of health issues at work, risk, and adjustments to the working environment. Large employers are likely to have this in house, others may commission it, or rely on information from hospital doctors or GPs.
- In the UK, the government employment service ('Jobcentre Plus') employs disability employment advisors, supported by occupational psychologists, who identify realistic job goals and training needs. They tend to become involved when return to the same job is not possible, but can also undertake interventions with employers to help retain disabled people in work. They may commission specialist vocational rehabilitation.
- Health professionals:
  - Clinical neuropsychologists assess potential cognitive barriers to work (or types of work), including attention, information processing, executive function, behaviour, emotion, and social skills, and devise therapy programmes to address difficulties.
  - Occupational therapists (especially in neurodisability and community rehabilitation services) can be central to the process, in both pre-work rehabilitation, and liaising with employers, negotiating adaptations or job-changes, and support during the return to work process. The availability or otherwise of an able and involved occupational therapist can make or break the process.

- Doctors may be called upon to provide reports on abilities and disabilities. These comprise findings on neurological examination, including any evidence of neglect, problems with proprioception and dexterity, and a cognitive assessment.
- Unions may also help with employer liaison.

Vocational rehabilitation comprises:
- Education about difficulties likely to affect work.
- Counselling to identify a suitable job.
- Development of skills/behaviours necessary for work, using material drawn from, or relevant to, the person's work.
- Restoring work-related routines (time-keeping, travel, money management).
- Building up attention, work tolerance and stamina ('work hardening').
- Learning coping strategies for use in the workplace.
- Assisted job selection, search, application, interviews.
- Voluntary work trials and supported work placements.

Employers are often worried about return to work. They need information, and may receive financial support, access to support workers, specialist aids and equipment, adaptations to premises or to existing equipment, and help with the additional costs of travel to work for people who are unable to use public transport.

In the UK, employers have obligations under the Disability Discrimination Act 1995, including keeping a job open, helping with return to work, and making 'reasonable adjustments' to enable continued employment. Line managers must understand the issues and have support if needed. Job modification may include changing the tasks duties or responsibilities of a job, use of special or adapted equipment, or change in site.

A return-to-work plan agreed between stakeholders might include:
- Graded return (supervised and gradual build-up of duties/hours).
- Initial informal return/voluntary trial basis.
- Short-term restrictions to duties/hours.
- Short-term flexibility (e.g. frequent breaks, variable hours, additional days off).
- Advice/support on implementing strategies in the workplace.
- Job coaching in the workplace.
- Additional support from colleagues in the workplace.
- Off-site support (e.g. from rehabilitation team).

Risk is best managed by initial close supervision, followed by progressive withdrawal as competence is demonstrated.

Care homes

Stroke, dementia, and hip fracture represent the 'big three' conditions leading to care home admission. There is remarkably little systematic work on the needs of stroke patients in care homes.

Care home residents are unstable: they are prone to deterioration due to recurrent stroke, complications (including polypharmacy and drug adverse effects), and intercurrent illness. Pressure sores and contractures are two particular complications that can develop quickly if care is suboptimal. However, care homes are also homes—they are not primarily therapeutic establishments. Occupation, diversion and activity, visiting by family and friends, and the process of care, including meals, become all the more important.

Ideally patients should not be permanently placed in a care home if there are outstanding rehabilitation needs. In the UK, at least, the provision of any sort of therapy in care homes is scant. However, given the prolonged time course of recovery, it is not unusual for functional gains to be made. This, and the need to maintain abilities and avoid complications, means that care home staff should adopt a 'rehabilitative approach', promoting or supporting independence in ADL, rather than simply delivering care to passive residents.

Summary

1. Patients and carers report many problems when they return home from hospital after a stroke, including those related to physical care of a disabled person, emotional responses, social limitations, financial problems, and difficulty in navigating a complex health and social care system when seeking help. 'Carer strain' is a problem in its own right.

2. The resettlement and readjustment elements of rehabilitation should address these, but they are often neglected. Community rehabilitation teams or family support workers can help. Training and education of carers also helps reduce psychological distress.

3. Fatigue is common and poorly understood. Exclude treatable medical or mental health causes, and encourage persisting with regular activity to prevent or reverse deconditioning. Recovery occurs over months or years.

4. A high-tone limb that is not carefully managed will develop problems. Self- or carer management is important in prevention. If problems are developing refer early to a specialist neurology or neurorehabilitation spasticity clinic for multidisciplinary management.

5. Aphasia also needs specialist long-term management and support, with approaches targeting impairment, compensation, adjustment, and carer support.

6. For those previously in paid work, voluntary work, or education, the issue of return to work should be addressed. Chances of successful return to work are greatly increased by careful assessment of neurological, cognitive, and psychological problems, job analysis, and a planned programme of communication with employers, identification of vocational rehabilitation needs, support, careful timing, and graded return.

Appendices

Appendix 1: Abbreviated Mental Test (AMT) score

Each item scores 1 point

1. Age.
2. Time (nearest hour).
3. Address (42 West Street).
4. Year.
5. Name of hospital.
6. Recognize two people.
7. Date of birth (month, year).
8. Year of First (or Second) World War.
9. Name of monarch.
10. Count backwards from 20–1.

Age and Ageing 1972; **1**:233–8.

Appendix 2: Mini-mental state examination, and Addenbrooke's Cognitive Examination

We are unable to reproduce the Mini Mental State Examination as it is copyrighted by Psychological Assessment Resources, Inc. The enforcement of this copyright is controversial, as it was originally distributed freely.

The MMSE is widely available in publications, on hospital wards, and may be found in the original publication (*Journal of Psychiatric Research* 1975, 12(3): 189-198). An internet search yields many examples of the full scale in pdf format. It is also described in Wikipedia (http://en.wikipedia.org/wiki/Mini-mental_state_examination).

It comprises 11 domains, dominated by attention and verbal memory:

- Orientation to place
- Orientation in time
- Registration
- Attention
- Recall
- Verbal understanding
- Written understanding
- Expressive language
- Repetition
- Syntax and writing
- Construction.

An expanded brief cognitive examination, the Addenbrooke's Cognitive Examination – Revised (ACE-R), incorporates the MMSE. This examines more cognitive domains than the MMSE, including verbal fluency, executive, and visuo-spatial functions. It also gives administration instructions and scoring conventions for all items, including the MMSE items.

It is freely available at http://pn.bmj.com/content/suppl/2007/07/19/7.4.245. DC1/74245app1.pdf.

Appendix 3: Glasgow Coma Scale

Best eye opening
- E1 none.
- E2 to pain.
- E3 to voice.
- E4 spontaneously with blinking.

Best motor response in unaffected limb
- M1 no response to pain.
- M2 arm extension to pain (decerebrate posturing).
- M3 arm flexion to pain (decorticate posturing).
- M4 arm withdraws from pain.
- M5 hand localizes pain.
- M6 obeys commands.

Best verbal response
- V1 none.
- V2 sounds, no recognizable words.
- V3 inappropriate words.
- V4 confused speech.
- V5 normal, orientated.

Lancet 1974; **ii**: 81.

Appendix 4: Days 1–3 nursing care pathway for stroke (Table A.1)

Table A.1 Day 1–3 nursing care pathway for stroke

Assessment	Action
Airway maintained	*If no:* recovery position, suction, oral airway
	If maintaining own airway: remove oral airway. Encourage coughing/chest physiotherapy
Check blood glucose	Inform doctor if initial level <3 or >10mmol/L. Monitor 1–2-hourly if on insulin sliding scale. Pre-meal and pre-bed if on other insulin regimen
Monitor oxygen saturation	Administer oxygen to keep SaO$_2$ >95%. Monitor 4-hourly
Temperature >37.5°C	Inform doctor. Give regular paracetamol. Obtain sputum and urine specimens. Monitor 4-hourly
Systolic blood pressure <140 or >200mmHg	Inform doctor. Assess conscious level and pain. Monitor 4-hourly
Pressure sore risk assessment	Appropriate pressure mattress/turning regimen
Record Scandinavian (or NIH) Stroke Scale	*If fallen > 5:* inform doctor. Decide monitoring frequency (twice daily unless informed otherwise)
Record GCS	*If fallen > 2:* inform doctor. Decide monitoring frequency (hourly 4-hourly unless informed otherwise)
Swallow safety	*If failed 3 screens:* refer speech and language therapy. Continue nil by mouth, IV fluids. Consider NG tube. Review route for medication
	Fluid balance chart. Mouth care. Discuss/review daily
	If safe: free fluids, normal diet
Altered diet required	Food chart. Dietician referral
IV cannula	Check site
Understanding of diagnosis	Discuss. Information booklets.
Moving and handling assessment, positioning plan	Allow to transfer or walk if clearly safe. Hoist if transfers unsafe. Neurological positioning. Refer physiotherapy. Assess need for bed rails (cot sides)
Continent of urine	*If no:* review, or complete assessment (urinalysis, PVRV bladder scan, 48-h output chart). Consider prompted voiding. Containment plan

Table A.1 (Contd.)

Assessment	Action
Continent of faeces	*If no:* review, or complete assessment (PR exam, bowel chart, specimen if diarrhoea). Containment plan
Communication problems	*If yes:* review. SLT referral if not too drowsy. Explain to relatives
Able to dress independently	*If no:* assist. Refer occupational therapy
Disability assessment	Pre-stroke and admission Barthel Index
Unable to sleep	*If yes:* assess why. Check position in bed. Check for pain and urinary symptoms. Medical assessment
Pain	*If yes:* assess, monitor. Give prescribed analgesics. Medical assessment
Is early discharge possible?	*If yes:* discuss with patient and family. Discuss with multidisciplinary team. Liaise with community rehabilitation service if needed

SaO$_2$, oxygen saturation; IV, intravenous; NG, nasogastric; PVRV, postvoid urinary residual volume; SLT speech and language therapy; PR per rectum.

Appendix 5: Thrombolysis work-up

- Cardiorespiratory assessment and resuscitation (adequate oxygenation, control of tachyarrhythmias and seizures, fluids for hypotension).
- Send blood urgently for FBC, urea and electrolytes, glucose, group and save serum. Request clotting studies (prothrombin time/INR, APTT), but do not wait for results if there is no reason to suspect an abnormality (i.e. recent warfarin or heparin). Urine for pregnancy test on women in whom pregnancy is possible.
- Arrange CT head scan.
- History, examination, including NIH stroke scale (15min maximum).
- BP monitoring:
  - Measure BP every 15–30min.
  - If it is >185/110mmHg do not thrombolyse unless it comes down spontaneously.
  - Some centres will attempt to reduce BP with IV drugs to 160–180/90–100mmHg (follow your local guidelines; see emergency BP control in next section).
- Complete suitability checklist (see 📖 Appendix 6, p.330).
- Consent (or assessment of best interests). Pre-written information sheet. Document discussions.

Emergency blood pressure control

For use after thrombolysis, in hypertensive encephalopathy, and other hypertensive emergencies.

- If diastolic BP >140mmHg, site an arterial line and give IV nitroprusside 0.5–10mcg/kg/min
- If systolic BP >230mmHg or diastolic BP 121–140mmHg, give labetalol 20mg IV over 2min then 10–20mg every 10–15min up to maximum 150mg (or IV labetalol infusion 2–8mg/min) until adequate response then discontinue.
- If systolic BP 180–230mmHg or diastolic BP 105–120mmHg give labetalol 10mg IV over 2min then 10–20mg every 10–15min up to maximum 150mg (or IV labetalol infusion 2–8mg/min) until adequate response then discontinue.
- If control inadequate, or beta-blockers contraindicated, site an arterial line and give IV nitroprusside.

Appendix 6: Suitability checklist for thrombolysis (Table A.2)

Table A.2 Suitability checklist for thrombolysis

Item	Criterion	Check
Onset	Time of onset known (time last known to be neurologically normal, time of first symptoms if subsequent progression, previous night if stroke present on waking up)	
Timing	Commencement of t-PA infusion possible within 4.5h	
Contraindications	Age within range 18–80 years	
	No history of severe uncontrolled hypertension	
	No bleeding disorder, including: No oral anticoagulants INR <1.4 No treatment-dose LMWH within 24h APTT normal if heparin within previous 48h Platelet count >100×10⁹/L	
	Blood sugar within range 2.8–22.2mmol/L	
	No major surgery, bleeding, or trauma in past 14 days	
	No previous ischaemic stroke or head injury within 3 months (excluding TIA with full recovery)	
	No history of any previous stroke if diabetic	
	No history of intracranial haemorrhage ever, including SAH, or symptoms of SAH even if CT normal	
	No history of structural CNS (including spinal) disease or surgery, including tumours, aneurysms or arteriovenous malformations	
	No diabetic retinopathy with new vessels	
	No peptic ulcer within past 3 months, oesophageal varices, severe liver disease, acute pancreatitis	

Table A.2 (Contd.)

Item	Criterion	Check
	No external cardiac massage, obstetric delivery, non-compressible arterial puncture, lumbar puncture or biopsies within 10 days (but not menstruation)	
	No endocarditis or pericarditis	
	No cancer with increased bleeding risk	
	Systolic BP <185 and diastolic <110mmHg	
	Pregnancy not possible (or pregnancy test negative)	
Stroke work-up	No seizure at onset	
	Neurological deficit present at least 30min	
	Neurological deficit not minor or rapidly improving	
	Not severe stroke (coma, NIH score >25)	
	Head scan performed and reported	
	No intracranial bleeding on head scan	
	Ischaemic stroke confirmed as likely diagnosis (mimics and bleeding excluded)	
Consent	Consent given (or assessment of best interests made). Information sheet given. Discussions documented	
Monitoring	High dependency bed available	

Appendix 7: Monitoring schedule for thrombolysis

Restrictions
- Bed rest for 24h.
- No urinary catheterization until at least 30min after infusion ends.
- Avoid nasogastric tube for 24h.
- No central venous access, arterial puncture, or intramuscular injections for 24h (except adrenaline for anaphylaxis).
- Nil by mouth for 24h except medication.
- No anticoagulants, aspirin, or non-steroidal anti-inflammatory drugs for 24h.

Monitoring
- High dependency bed for 24h.
- Vital signs, and neurological observations (GCS, arm /leg weakness):
  - Every 15min for 1h before and 2h after starting infusion.
  - Every 30min for 6h.
  - Hourly until 24h after starting infusion.
- Confirm neurological deterioration by repeating full NIHSS (deterioration is ≥4 points).
- Arrange a CT immediately if there is neurological deterioration.
- Arrange a follow up CT after 24–36h, before aspirin or anticoagulants are given.

Intervention
- BP—maintain below 185mmHg systolic and 110mmHg diastolic using IV drugs for 24h.
- Look for overt bleeding and give more IV fluids if BP drops below 140/80mmHg.
- Anaphylactoid reactions may occur (in 1.5%; hypotension, bronchospasm, urticaria, rash, angio-oedema). Stop tPA infusion. Continue oxygen, give more IV fluids, chlorphenamine 10mg IV, hydrocortisone 200mg IV. If severe breathing problems or hypotension give adrenaline (500mcg = 0.5mL of 1/1000 solution IM, repeated if necessary every 5min).
- If level of consciousness or symptoms worsen, new headache or vomiting, or acute blood pressure rise, stop tPA infusion. Repeat CT head scan immediately. Check FBC, fibrinogen, and clotting. Consult a haematologist urgently. Give fibrinogen concentrate (or cryoprecipitate), and platelets, if <100 × 10⁹/L.
- Skin, gum, and nose bleeding usually do not require action.
- If other bleeding occurs, stop tPA infusion. Most patients can be managed with fluid replacement. If deterioration continues, continue fluid resuscitation, give fibrinogen/ cryoprecipitate, fresh frozen plasma/ prothrombin complex concentrate, and platelets on the advice of a haematologist. Check clotting and fibrinogen after each administration, target fibrinogen 1–2g/L.

Appendix 8: NIH stroke scale (Table A.3)

Detailed administration guidelines available at 🕫 http://www.ninds.nih.gov/doctors/NIH_Stroke_Scale.pdf

Table A.4 NIH stroke scale

Function	Score	Description
Level of consciousness responsiveness	0	Fully alert, immediately responsive
	1	Drowsy, arouses to voice or shaking, and responds appropriately
	2	Stuporous; aroused with difficulty, needs painful stimulus; lapses back when unstimulated
	3	Comatose, unresponsive to all stimuli
LOC orientation	0	Knows own age, and correct month *on initial answer. No coaching*
	1	Answers one question correctly (or intubated, severely dysarthric or language barrier)
	2	Unable to answer either question (including aphasic and stuporous patients)
LOC commands	0	Opens/closes (non-paretic) hand, and closes/opens eyes to command
	1	Does one correctly
	2	Does neither correctly
Best gaze	0	Normal
	1	Partial gaze palsy (overcome by voluntary or reflex movement)
	2	Forced deviation; total gaze paresis not overcome by oculocephalic (doll's eyes) manoeuvre
Visual fields	0	Normal (upper and lower quadrants)
	1	Partial hemianopia/quadrantanopia
	2	Complete hemianopia
	3	Bilateral hemianopia (or blind from any cause)

Table A.3 (Contd.)

Function	Score	Description
Facial palsy	0	Normal
	1	Minor asymmetry with smiling and speech, but good volitional movement
	2	Partial: definite weakness but some movement remains
	3	Complete (including comatose, bilateral and lower motor neuron weakness)
Right arm—test for drift at 90° for 10s (count out loud)	0	No drift
	1	Drift; some fluttering
	2	Some effort against gravity but unable to keep arm up for all 10s
	3	No effort against gravity but muscle movement present
	4	No movement
Left arm	0	No drift
	1	Drift; some fluttering
	2	Some effort against gravity but unable to keep arm up for all 10s
	3	No effort against gravity but muscle movement present
	4	No movement
Right leg—test lifting to 30° for 5s (count out loud)	0	No drift
	1	Drift; some fluttering
	2	Some effort against gravity but unable to keep arm up for all 5s
	3	No effort against gravity but muscle movement present
	4	No movement
Left leg	0	No drift
	1	Drift; some fluttering
	2	Some effort against gravity but unable to keep arm up for all 5s
	3	No effort against gravity but muscle movement present
	4	No movement

Table A.3 (Contd.)

Function	Score	Description
Limb ataxia (out of proportion to weakness)	0	Normal (finger–nose and heel–shin tests) or too weak to test
	1	Present unilaterally in either arm or leg
	2	Present unilaterally in both arm and leg, or bilaterally
Sensory—tested with pin/pain (not hands or feet)	0	Normal
	1	Mild: pinprick less sharp, patient aware of being tested
	2	Severe: patient unaware of being tested (including coma)
Language— aphasia testing (naming, describing picture)	0	Normal language
	1	Mild to moderate aphasia; word finding errors, naming errors, paraphrasias, mild impairment of communication either by comprehension or expression disability
	2	Severe aphasia: fully developed expressive or receptive aphasia
	3	Mute or global aphasia (or coma)
Dysarthria (give sentence list)	0	Normal articulation
	1	Mild to moderate dysarthria: patient has problems with articulation with mild to moderate slurring of words. The patient can be understood
	2	Near unintelligible or worse (or mute or unresponsive)
Neglect—testing the ability to recognize simultaneous stimuli of sensation and vision	0	No neglect; can recognize double sensory cutaneous stimulation and able to identify images in both visual fields simultaneously
	1	Partial neglect: unable to recognize both stimuli simultaneously for either cutaneous or visual
	2	Complete neglect: unable to recognize both stimuli for both cutaneous and visual

Appendix 9: Scandinavian Stroke Scale (Table A.4)

Table A.4 Scandinavian Stroke Scale

Function	Score	Description
Consciousness	6	Fully conscious
	4	Somnolent, can be awaked to full consciousness
	2	Reacts to verbal command, but is not fully conscious
	0	Unresponsive to verbal command
Eye movement	4	No gaze palsy
	2	Gaze palsy present
	0	Conjugate eye deviation
Arm, motor power, affected side	6	Raises arm with normal strength
	5	Raises arm with reduced strength
	4	Raises arm with flexion in elbow
	2	Can move, but not against gravity
	0	Paralysis
Hand, motor power, affected side	6	Normal strength
	4	Reduced strength in full range
	2	Some movement, fingertips do not reach palm
	0	Paralysis
Leg, motor power, affected side	6	Normal strength
	5	Raises straight leg with reduced strength
	4	Raises leg with flexion of knee
	2	Can move, but not against gravity
	0	Paralysis
Orientation	6	Correct for time, place, and person
	4	Two of these
	2	One of these
	0	Completely disorientated

Table A.4 *(Contd.)*

Function	Score	Description
Speech	10	No aphasia
	6	Limited vocabulary or incoherent speech
	3	More than yes/no but not longer sentences
	0	Only yes/no or less
Facial palsy	2	None/dubious
	0	Present
Gait	12	Walks 5m without aids
	9	Walks with aids
	6	Walks with help of another person
	3	Sits without support
	0	Bedridden/wheelchair

Appendix 10: Care pathway for urinary continence assessment and management

1. Complete within a week of admission.
2. Document history of continence problems and lower urinary tract symptoms (urgency, frequency, dysuria, nocturia, poor stream, hesitancy).
3. Consider non-bladder factors which may affect continence:
   - Functional:
     - Mobility.
     - Aphasia.
     - Language.
     - Visuospatial problems.
     - Drowsiness.
     - Dementia or delirium.
     - Dexterity.
   - Environmental:
     - Distance to toilet.
     - Privacy.
     - Ability to reach aid.
     - Equipment available.
     - Staff available.
   - Behavioural:
     - Current medication.
     - Ability to recognize cues.
     - Ability to recognize toilet.
     - Inhibitions.
     - Depression.
     - Motivation.
4. Commence 48-h fluid balance/frequency–volume chart. Identify functional bladder capacity (largest void), number of voids day/night, total volume passed day/night.
5. Urinalysis, and culture if positive.
6. Exclude incomplete bladder emptying (bladder scan) and faecal impaction.
7. Identify diagnoses:
   - Faecal impaction (laxatives).
   - Urinary infection (antibiotics, cranberry juice, avoid catheter, exclude incomplete emptying, image upper urinary tracts if male or recurrent, topical oestrogen).
   - Nocturnal polyuria (check glycosuria, calcium, oedema, heart failure, renal function, consider daytime diuretics or desmopressin).
   - Bladder instability (increase fluids, reduce caffeine, bladder training, pelvic floor exercises, anticholinergic drugs).
   - Stress incontinence (pelvic floor exercises, cones, electrotherapy, biofeedback).

- Outflow obstruction—consider benign prostatic hyperplasia or carcinoma, stricture (alpha-blocker, finasteride, refer urology).
- Hypocontractility (stop anticholinergic drugs, try alpha-blocker, bladder stimulator, intermittent catheter, indwelling catheter).
- Drug side effects (review diuretics, anticholinergic drugs).
- Atrophic urethritis (topical oestrogen).

8. Consider prompted voiding ('regular toileting').
9. Optimize containment—pads, sheath catheter.

Appendix 11: Rivermead Motor Assessment

Each item is scored 1 (succeed) or 0 (fail)

- Sit, feet unsupported 10s.
- Lying to sitting on side of bed.
- Sit to standing in 15s for 15s.
- Transfer from chair to chair towards unaffected side.
- Transfer from chair to chair towards affected side.
- Walk 10m independently with an aid.
- Climb stairs, may use a banister.
- Walk 10m independently without an aid.
- Walk 5m, pick up a bean bag from floor and return.
- Walk outside 40m (with aid if required).
- Walk up and down 4 steps (no banister or wall support).
- Run 10m in 4s.
- Hop on affected leg 5 times on the spot.

Appendix 12: The Barthel Index (Table A.5)

Table A.5 The Barthel Index

Activity	Criterion	Score
Continence of urine	Continent	2
	Wet less than once a day	1
	Wet once a day or more, or catheter	0
Continence of faeces	Continent	2
	Soils less than once a week	1
	Soils more than once a week (or given enemas)	0
Toilet use	Independent (including clothes and wiping)	2
	Needs some help	1
	Unable or full help	0
Transfers (bed–chair)	Independent	3
	Minor help (help of one)	2
	Major help (can sit, needs one or two)	1
	Unable (cannot stand)	0
Walking (on the flat, using any aid)	Independent (at least 10m)	3
	Needs human help	2
	Wheelchair independent (including round corners)	1
	Unable	0
Feeding	Independent	2
	Help cutting up, buttering bread	1
	Unable	0
Dressing	Independent (including buttons, zips, laces)	2
	Manages half	1
	Unable	0

Table A.5 *(Contd.)*

Activity	Criterion	Score
Grooming (teeth, hair, shaving, wash face)	Independent	1
	Needs help	0
Using bath or shower	Independent	1
	Needs help	0
Stairs	Independent	2
	Needs help (verbal/physical/carrying aid)	1
	Unable	0

Appendix 13: Framingham risk scores (Tables A.6–A.8)

Overall risk scores for stroke among men and women who are not in AF (*Stroke* 1994; **25**:40–3).

Table A.6 Risk score for men aged 55–85 years

Risk score	0	+1	+2	+3	+4	+5	+6	+7	+8	+9	+10
						Points					
Age, years	54–56	57–59	60–62	63–65	66–68	69–72	73–75	76–78	79–81	82–84	85
Untreated SBP, mmHg	97–105	106–115	116–125	126–135	136–145	146–155	156–165	166–175	176–185	186–195	196–205
Treated SBP, mmHg	97–105	106–112	113–117	118–123	124–129	130–135	136–142	143–150	151–161	162–176	177–205
Diabetes	No		Yes								
Current smoker	No			Yes							
CVD	No				Yes						
ECG LVH	No					Yes					

Table A.7 Risk score for women aged 55–85 years

Risk score	0	+1	+2	+3	+4	+5	+6	+7	+8	+9	+10
						Points					
Age, years	54–56	57–59	60–62	63–64	65–67	68–70	71–73	74–76	77–78	79–81	82–84
Untreated SBP, mmHg		95–106	107–118	119–130	131–143	144–155	156–167	168–180	181–192	193–204	205–216
Treated SBP, mmHg		95–106	107–113	114–119	20–125	136–131	32–139	140–148	149–160	161–204	205–216
Diabetes	No			Yes							
Current smoker	No			Yes							
CVD	No		Yes								
LVH	No				Yes						

SBP, systolic BP; CVD, cardiovascular disease (history of MI, angina, intermittent claudication, heart failure); LVH, left ventricular hypertrophy on ECG

Table A.8 Conversion of points derived from risk factor profiles to probability of stroke over 10 years

Points	10-year probability, men (%)	10-year probability, women (%)	Points	10-year probability, men (%)	10-year probability, women (%)	Points	10-year probability, men (%)	10-year probability, women (%)
1	3	1	11	11	8	21	42	43
2	3	1	12	13	9	22	47	50
3	4	2	13	15	11	23	52	57
4	4	2	14	14	13	24	57	64
5	5	2	15	20	16	25	63	71
6	5	3	16	22	19	26	68	78
7	6	4	17	26	23	27	74	84
8	7	4	18	29	27	28	79	
9	8	5	19	33	32	29	84	
10	10	6	20	37	37	30	88	

Appendix 14: Risk of stroke in atrial fibrillation—Framingham risk profile (Tables A.9 and Fig. A.1)

(Excluding rheumatic mitral stenosis, who should all be considered at high risk; people on warfarin; and people within 30 days of going into AF). *Journal of the American Medical Association* 2003; **290**:1049–56.

Excel spreadsheet available at ✆ http://www.nhlbi.nih.gov/about/framingham/stroke.htm

Table A.9 Risk score for stroke in AF

Risk score	0	+1	+2	+3	+4	+5	+6	+7	+8	+9	+10
Age, years	54–59	60–62	63–66	67–71	72–74	75–77	78–81	82–85	86–90	91–93	>93
Sex	Male						Female				
SBP, mmHg	<120	120–139	140–159	160–179	>179						
Diabetes	No					Yes					
Prior stroke or TIA	No						Yes				

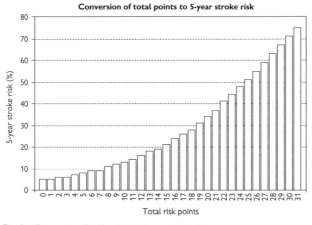

Fig. A1 Conversion of total points to 5-year stroke risk.
Data from *JAMA* 2003; **290**:1049–105.

Index